Demystifying Prostatitis

Words of Wisdom

from A Prostate Specialist

Ilia Kaploun

DEMYSTIFYING PROSTATITIS

Copyright © 2020 Ilia Kaploun
All rights reserved.

This book, or parts thereof, may not be reproduced in any form without the express written permission of the author.

This publication is designed to provide information with regard to the subject matter covered. It is sold with the understanding that the author and publisher are not engaged in rendering legal, accounting or other professional advice. If legal advice or other expert assistance is required, the services of a competent professional should be sought.

ISBN: 9798669679835

TABLE OF CONTENTS

FOREWORD i

DEMYSTIFYING PROSTATITIS
Practical Wisdom from a Prostate Specialist v

CHAPTER 1
Walnut or Peach? 1

CHAPTER 2
Sorry guys… Science is boring, but please stick around for this one …… 5

CHAPTER 3
What came first: The Chicken or the Egg? 11

CHAPTER 4
What makes men miserable and why? 19

CHAPTER 5
That time you have problems in the bedroom, and it isn't the snoring .. 31

CHAPTER 6
To Ejaculate or Not to Ejaculate, that is the question! 45

CHAPTER 7
Does size matter? 53

CHAPTER 8
The biggest fear of all: Cancer 61

CHAPTER 9
How do you like your Head - With the Helmet or Without? 69

CHAPTER 10
Sorry if you love beer 75

CHAPTER 11
How expensive can pee really get? 95

IN CONCLUSION
Do I get used to it or Do something about it? 105

ACKNOWLEDGEMENTS 109

REFERENCES 111

DEMYSTIFYING PROSTATITIS

FOREWORD

It is an honour to have been asked to write a forward for this very timely and important book on chronic prostatitis.

Prostatitis is not well understood by most people and many doctors. People generally don't appreciate how much of an impact prostatitis has on men's lives and don't feel that prostatitis is as important as some of the other medical problems ("at least you don't have prostate cancer"). But…prostatitis is very common, has a significant adverse effect on the lives of men and their families and is often overlooked and undertreated.

It is also challenging for men to discuss prostatitis with family, friends and health care professionals. This is understandable, since the condition is poorly understood and many men find it embarrassing to discuss the pain or problems they have "down there".

For most people the prostate and all of the other "things" in that area are not well understood, the diseases affecting the area even more mysterious and for most, how to prevent/treat prostate diseases is doubly mysterious.

A book on "demystifying prostatitis" provides a public service to men of all ages who want to understand more about prostatitis and how they might prevent or treat this condition. I can think of no one better than Ilia Kaploun to write such a book.

I have had the pleasure to work with Ilia at the Mount Sinai Hospital for the past 18 years (it seems scary to think that we have known each other this long). Ilia's life work has been to educate men about prostatitis, treat men with prostatitis and prevent men from developing prostatitis. Ilia is the third generation of Kaplouns studying and working on prostatitis. I am sure that he grew up talking and thinking about prostatitis. He has not stopped talking and

DEMYSTIFYING PROSTATITIS

thinking about prostatitis ever since I have known him. His passion to understand and treat men with prostatitis continues unchecked.

I hope this book helps men of all ages understand this common problem, but also helps to normalize conversations about prostatitis. This should allow men with prostatitis to talk more openly about their problems with family and friends and seek health care earlier.

I would like to thank Ilia for all of the time and effort he took to write this book and congratulate him on producing a highly informative but easy to read publication.

Keith Jarvi, MD FRCSC
Chief, Division of Urology, Mount Sinai Hospital,
Professor, Dept. Of Surgery, University of Toronto

DEDICATION

I dedicate this book to my true hero, my father.

Thank you, father, for inspiring me to write this book. Thank you for all the knowledge, wisdom, and dedication you instilled into my heart and soul. I hope this book makes you proud of me.

I also would like to dedicate this book to my brother. I have an older brother who is also a urologist successfully practising in Israel. His expertise focuses on female urology. I remember years ago he did research on Paraurethral Syndrome. Interesting enough, it is another mysterious condition which affects many women and often referred to as "Female Prostatitis". Unfortunately, due to life circumstances we have been living worlds apart for many years. Nevertheless, there is not a day goes by when I do not think about him and his family. I look up to him when it comes to professional life. I am incredibly grateful to him for looking after our parents for so many years. I really hope that he will appreciate this book and make him feel proud of his younger brother.

DEMYSTIFYING PROSTATITIS

DEMYSTIFYING PROSTATITIS
Practical Wisdom from a Prostate Specialist

Preface

My family has three generations of urologists. My grandfather was a urologist, my father was a urologist and my brother, and I are urologists. I doubt that there are many other families who can claim the same professional lineage within this stream of medicine.

To provide you with a bit of background, my father dedicated most of his professional life to researching and treating Prostatitis but he never had a professional title beyond being a practicing urologist. He was one of the top experts on Prostatitis in the former Soviet Union and published many research papers in leading Urology peer review journals. Many of his articles were requested by American and European Urologists specializing in Prostatitis. He has treated many patients from all over the country and I deeply admired him. I watched him come home, exhausted after spending long and difficult workdays in the operating room. After eating his supper, he would go into his "office," retrieve his typewriter, and start typing his essays about Prostatitis. He would write for hours. Eventually, after failing to defend his PhD thesis due to Moscow politics, he published a book on this same subject: "Chronic Prostatitis". It is quite fascinating how politics play out in science, research and medicine. I do not think it is necessarily only a Russian phenomenon. Politics are everywhere. They permeate the professional field around the world. But I believe that politics in the former Soviet Union have been subject to a higher level of corruption. My father's thesis supervisor was a Chief Urologist of the Russian state, but to defend a PhD level thesis in urology someone had to submit their work to a Chief Urologist of the Soviet Union. The problem there was that the Chief Urologists of the

DEMYSTIFYING PROSTATITIS

Soviet Union were not overly fond of the Chief Urologist of the Russian state. As a result, every applicant under a Chief Urologist of a Russian state had failed. Knowing this, my father decided to spare himself the grief of going under such stress just to be told at the end that he did not pass, and he instead decided to publish his thesis as a textbook. Ever since, his book became my "bible", guide in mastering the art of prostatitis management.

From this, I inherited his keen interest in this mysterious condition. I have spent many years assessing and treating men suffering from Chronic Prostatitis (CP). My desire to learn more on this subject has never stopped. Though I keep searching for new information in scientific periodicals, the volume of research on this subject is very low. Astonishingly, there is very little interest in CP among urologists in Western medicine and sadly, there is practically zero interest in the private sector in investing in research on CP. This is particularly appalling because the need is enormous. There are millions of men all over the world who suffer from this condition, and many of them have a severe form of CP, which significantly affects their quality of life.

Thank you, father, for inspiring me to write this book. Thank you for all the knowledge, wisdom and dedication you instilled into my heart and soul. I hope this book makes you proud of me.

I would also like to thank all of my patients - past, present and future - who have entrusted me with their pain and suffering, and most importantly, their prostate health - and who travel relentlessly with me along the often challenging path towards healing.

On a lighter note, these brave patients gave me their prostates (or at least lent them) to my trusty index finger, which has probably probed more prostates over the years than any other finger in North America and

DEMYSTIFYING PROSTATITIS

beyond. Come to think of it, I really should be donating that skillful index finger - my legacy - to humanity as a beacon of hope for future generations of men who need a caring urologist.

Finally, this is why I decided to write this book. I want my readers to have access to information that is easy to understand about prostatitis and related conditions such as prostate enlargement, prostate cancer, sexual dysfunction, and chronic pelvic pain syndrome. I want to empower my readers with this knowledge so that they can adjust their lifestyles in order to improve their overall quality of life. There is a lot of information about this subject all over the internet in chat groups, blogs, and articles, and although it is easy to access and predominantly free, unfortunately a lot of this information is misleading or false. As a result, many men develop severe anxieties and suffer enormous stress, which diminishes their quality of life, triggers family discord and negatively affects their ability to work. So, in this book I have compiled my scientific based knowledge and my personal experience of having treated hundreds of patients over the last 20 years to bring you a comprehensive source of information where patients can get as many answers as possible in order to minimize stress and fear of the unknown.

This book by no means replaces any medical advice from your doctor. You should always seek help from your medical professional. Additionally, this book is not intended to be a scientific publication for medical professionals (although they may want to recommend this book to patients with prostate issues!).

So, please make sure that when you read this book you are either sitting on a comfortable chair, couch, or maybe lying down. Or better yet, walking on a treadmill. Enjoy your read and get ready to find the answers to the many questions you may have about prostate-related health issues.

DEMYSTIFYING PROSTATITIS

CHAPTER 1

Walnut or Peach?

Dear readers, let me take you on a short excursion into the anatomy of the male pelvis, the very topic of this book.

My patients often ask me to describe what the prostate looks like and to tell them the size of their own prostate. This isn't easy because no two prostates are alike. When it comes to depicting size, the best analogy would be to compare the prostate to the size of certain fruit or nuts. The prostate is one of the organs in the human body that can be readily compared to food products. Yes, we do compare kidneys to beans when it comes to shape, but not size.

So, if we take a young man, say between the ages of 16 and 40, we can compare the prostate to the size of a walnut. If we move past the age of 40, the fruits come into play. Unfortunately, as we get older, the prostate grows bigger. This is called an Enlarged Prostate (BPH - Benign Prostatic Hyperplasia). For example, a plum can progress into a peach and then possibly an orange or a grapefruit. We will talk about BPH in a separate chapter.

Let's stick to walnuts for now.

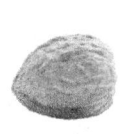

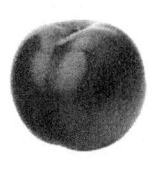

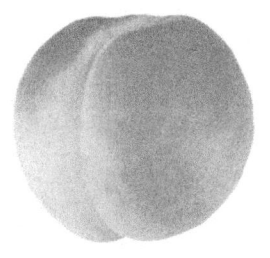

At the risk of boring you, I am going to describe this part of the male anatomy in some detail because all these components play an integral part in prostatitis as a medical condition.

DEMYSTIFYING PROSTATITIS

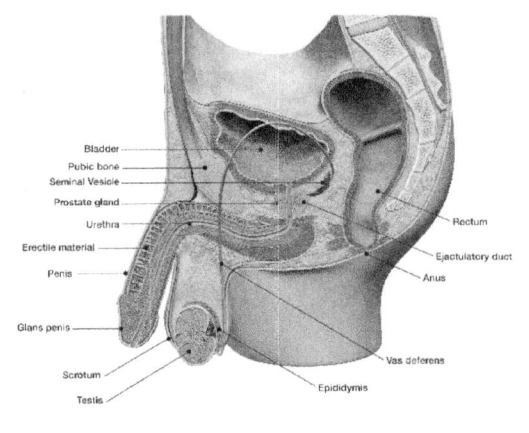

Anatomically, the prostate is conveniently located beneath the bladder, wrapping a portion of the urethra which connects to the bladder. The urethra is a tube which stretches from the bladder through the penis and exits at the tip of the penis (Glans Penis). The opening is called the Meatus. The prostate partially envelopes the urethra, which makes this area intimately entangled. The prostate, urethra and bladder opening (bladder neck), and the set of various muscles surrounding these organs, make up this area.

Next, we cannot forget the seminal vesicles which extend from the prostate and conveniently position themselves above the prostate and behind the bladder. The seminal vesicles' hidden secret is the so-called "Seminal Fluid", which makes up most of the volume of semen that men produce during ejaculation.

There are also testicles, located in a scrotal sac away from our troubled prostate. They are responsible for most of the testosterone production which makes men, well, "men". The testicles also produce spermatozoids, which help make babies. We are not going to pay too much attention to testicles. They are a subject of interest to fertility specialists but, honestly, have little relevance to our topic of interest.

Our next logical question then would be, "What does the prostate look like on the inside?" To answer that question, we can move on to vegetable comparisons.

I think the best way to describe the inside of a prostate is like the head of a broccoli. The prostate is a gland. It contains hundreds of microscopic sized glands called acini. Each acinus secretes a small amount of fluid we call Prostatic Secretion (PS). This PS then flows through tiny ducts into bigger ducts and eventually finds itself in the portion of the urethra located inside the prostate. Under "normal" circumstances, when men are just relaxing, working at their desks or hunting a moose, PS quietly sits within the acini. Once men become excited, let's say by watching hockey, baseball, Game of Thrones, or when they become sexually aroused, the prostate starts to produce more of its fluid under the influence of testosterone. And finally, when men reach orgasm all three components - spermatozoids, seminal fluid from the seminal vesicles, and prostatic secretion - get mixed together inside the prostatic portion of the urethra and with the help of all the muscles in the prostate, seminal vesicles and surrounding muscles, it is all forced outward, into the outside world.

Another commonly asked question is, "Why do we need a prostate?"

The simplest answer is because the prostate helps the sperm make babies. That's it, that's all. Men who have their prostates removed, continue to live completely normal and healthy lives. Often, they even preserve their normal sexual performance, but no semen is being produced on orgasm, because their seminal vesicles have been removed at the same time. It's as simple as that! So, it would seem that there is no vital importance that originates from this walnut or peach or grapefruit gland - especially in comparison to our other organs, including the neighbouring bladder. So then how can it inflict so much misery in men who suffer from prostatitis?

I wish I had an answer.

We will be talking about the symptoms of prostatitis and it's many root causes, but it must first be acknowledged that much is still unknown about this organ. A lot of research is being conducted about prostate cancer, some on prostate enlargement (BPH), but very, very little on prostatitis. Our knowledge about prostatitis now is almost the same as what was known 10 years ago. Honestly, I truly believe that

DEMYSTIFYING PROSTATITIS

my father knew more about prostatitis 40 years ago, than many specialists in Western countries now.

And with that, we have reached the climax of our lesson on the size and role of the prostate in the healthy male. Without further ado, we can now begin Demystifying Prostatitis.

CHAPTER 2

Sorry guys... Science is boring, but please stick around for this one...

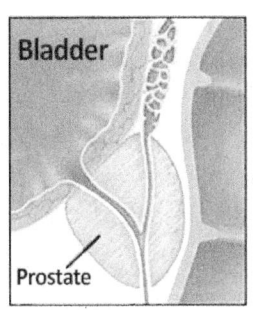

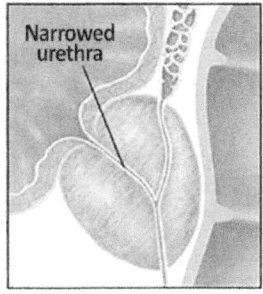

"Prostatitis", in its simplified definition, means "inflamed prostate". It has nothing to do with size. I often receive phone calls from men in their 60's and 70's (God bless them all) who think they have prostatitis but once we start discussing their problems, it appears they have problems related to prostate enlargement instead. Many of them even carry long term urinary catheters because they cannot pee. This could be caused by prostate enlargement or prostate cancer but not prostatitis.

We usually divide prostatitis into two categories: acute and chronic. The majority of men suffer from chronic prostatitis.

Chronic Prostatitis (CP)

Some of my patients, during their first visit, complain about a variety of prostate-related symptoms, which started only a few weeks before they sat down in my office. These men look fine, talking, walking, peeing and working. When I tell them that their concerns are due to a flare up of chronic prostatitis, most look totally surprised. "How?", and "Why?" they ask. And, here is where a small lecture begins, starting with a discussion on acute prostatitis...

DEMYSTIFYING PROSTATITIS

Acute Prostatitis (AP)

When a man develops acute prostatitis, he will become very sick. He will experience high fever, body aches, sometimes severe pain in the lower pelvic area (including the area between the scrotum and the rectum), and frequent but poor urination. Often, men cannot urinate at all because their prostate swells up, thus blocking the exit of urine from the bladder. Acute prostatitis often requires an **urgent trip** to the nearest Emergency Room for assessment and treatment or a visit to your general practitioner. It is almost always caused by some type of bad bacteria and thus, requires antibiotic treatment. Hopefully they get a long enough course of antibiotics so that their acute prostatitis does not evolve into chronic prostatitis.

Now, let's get back to chronic prostatitis. As I mentioned above, prostatitis means "inflamed prostate". Inflammation often causes a variety of symptoms. What are the symptoms of prostatitis? I usually divide them into a few categories:

General or Systemic:

When men experience a flare up of prostatitis they often complain about fatigue, malaise, occasional chills, nausea, lack of drive to do anything, anxiety and depression. In some cases, they put their entire lives on hold.

For example, I have had patients who have postponed their marriage proposals because they felt so down. I have had young men who were determined to be cured for their weddings three or four months away. They just wanted to get better before taking any future big steps in their lives. Can you imagine the emotional pressure they placed on themselves and their partners?

Sound depressing? Yes, it does, but there is a light at the end of the tunnel. Cheer up guys, I promise everything will be OK.

DEMYSTIFYING PROSTATITIS

Local Symptoms

Is it all in my head or is it real and will I suffer this pain, discomfort and these nagging sensations for the rest of my life?...

Please imagine a young man, let's say in his 30s', visiting his doctor more than once with the same symptoms. His doctor does a urine test, which shows nothing abnormal. The doctor may say:

It may be prostatitis...

I don't know...

Go see a Urologist...

It's all in your head...

Which words were most appealing to you?

Let's say you end up going to see a Urologist. Many experienced urologists will, after speaking with you about your symptoms, perform a procedure called a cystoscopy, which is when a thin flexible tube with a camera and light on the end is (very carefully) inserted into the urethra at the tip of the penis. The cystoscope travels all the way to the prostate area and into the bladder. Most men, especially younger ones, will be reassured that the cystoscopy was completely normal. There is absolutely nothing to worry about. Moreover, not much can be done about this condition and, therefore, hopefully this problem will go away on its own. Just get used to it and hope for the best.

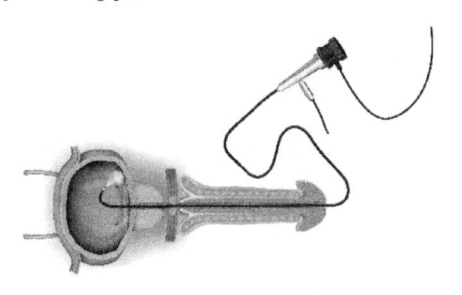

So, allow me, for the sake of completeness, to review all of the symptoms men with CP may, or may not, experience. Please remember, **you do not need to "get used to it"**. This is a condition

DEMYSTIFYING PROSTATITIS

which can and must be treated. So, please cheer up and browse this list...

Most men complain about:

Pain symptoms:

- Pain and discomfort in the groin, along the penile shaft and/or stinging at the tip of the penis:
- Lower back pain.
- Pain in the perineal area (between the bottom of the scrotum and anal area).
- Pain sometimes radiating down the hips.
- Pain in the lower pelvic area (bladder area).
- Pain in the scrotum

As you can see from the list above, pain or discomfort can be anywhere in the pelvic region. Many men complain about a "golf ball" pain in the perineal area because they feel like they are sitting on one.

Urinary symptoms:

- Urinary urgency (feeling like you have to pee right now) and frequency (endless trips to the bathroom).
- Sensation of incomplete bladder emptying.
- Stop & Go urination (interrupted urination).
- Weak stream (worse than your father's).
- Burning on urination.
- Excessive dribbling after urinating (don't you hate that wet feeling on your leg after your pants are up?).

Sexual problems:

- Difficulty getting and maintaining an erection.
- Low sexual desire.

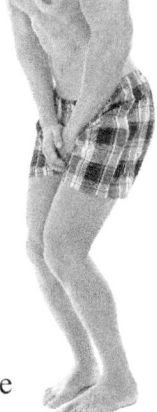

DEMYSTIFYING PROSTATITIS

- Premature ejaculation (climaxing much sooner than you want to and used to).
- Pain/burning during or after ejaculation.
- Weaker force of ejaculation.
- Reduced sensation of climax.
- Seminal fluid changed in volume, consistency or discoloration.
- Signs of blood in semen.

Please, if you experience severe symptoms of any kind, <u>seek medical help immediately</u>.

As you can see, my dear readers, CP can present itself with a vast variety of symptoms. I have had patients who have had them all. Most men will have some.

You can pretty much mix and match them but in the end, there is a good chance that a person with at least some of the above symptoms has Chronic Prostatitis.

Oh, I totally forgot to mention one very important detail...

Did you know that CP is one of the **most common health problems in men between the ages of 18 and 60**? It is estimated that between 10 and 15% of all men in the world suffer from CP at least once in their lifetimes [1,2,3,4,5].

It is also important to know that CP does not discriminate by race, or social status. Men from all over the world, all walks of life suffer from this condition.

What is known to improve your chances of a cure? Access to health care and education. You need to know everything about CP in order to know how to deal with it. This book will help you to acquire just that.

And if it makes you feel any better, you are not alone. You do not need to suffer in silence. Talk to those close to you: your wives, partners, parents and close friends. Share your emotions with whomever you feel most comfortable. It will make your life so much

DEMYSTIFYING PROSTATITIS

easier. You need emotional support from your loved ones as much as you need physical support from your medical experts. Often you need financial support too. Unfortunately, this book may not directly provide you with either physical or financial support, but it will provide you with knowledge and emotional support.

Our demystification of prostatitis goes on…

CHAPTER 3

What came first: The Chicken or the Egg?

Here we have finally reached a climactic point in my book: Chronic Prostatitis - causes, types and pitfalls.

Let's take an example:

A young man - let's name him John, age 35, married with two children. John suddenly starts to experience a nagging, burning pain in his groin behind the scrotum, urinary frequency, urinary urgency and burning on urination. He has also started to notice that his erections are not as strong as they used to be, and there is discomfort along the penile shaft after ejaculation.

John is obviously upset. He does not know what's going on. He Googles his symptoms. It seems like they point toward prostatitis. John goes to see his family doctor, who talks to him and collects a urine sample for urinalysis and culture. John returns to his doctor four days later, still complaining about the same symptoms. His doctor reports that the urine tests came back normal but decides to prescribe an antibiotic because the symptoms are indicative of prostatitis. He prescribes a 7-10 day course of Ciprofloxacin. John goes home somewhat relieved with his doctor's reassurance. He starts taking Cipro, and behold, 3-4 days later his symptoms are drastically reduced. Everything points to a full cure. John is happy, finishes his treatment and carries on with his life.

Suddenly, two weeks later, his symptoms return.

He goes back to his family doctor, who performs a quick prostate exam.

DEMYSTIFYING PROSTATITIS

What is he going to do now? He refers John to a urologist, and in the meantime, prescribes Ciprofloxacin for four weeks.

A few weeks later, he sees the Urologist while continuing to present the same symptoms, which diminish somewhat and then flare up again. The Urologist decides to perform a cystoscopy. What does he/she see there? Actually, in many cases, nothing abnormal. Sometimes there's an inflammation of the prostate. The urologist tells John that he most likely has nonbacterial chronic prostatitis, which will gradually go away by itself within some period of time.

There are variations in responses. Some urologists may prescribe even more Cipro, or another antibiotic. Some will prescribe some kind of anti-inflammatory drug.

I have seen so many men over the years who went through exactly this scenario.

So, what is really happening? Why is it so difficult to diagnose prostatitis? What causes prostatitis? Is it an infection? Is it just stress and lifestyle related? Is there something else we don't know about?

The answer is...are you ready? ALL OF THE ABOVE. Wow! A great multiple-choice answer. There is a reason why chronic prostatitis is called the "Waste Basket" of clinical ignorance[6,7]. There are so many layers to prostatitis. What do we get with Prostatitis? Pain, endless peeing and bad sex. I hear you my dear readers!

I have treated so many men with extremely complicated issues related to prostatitis. Every time I hear a complicated story in my office, even when symptoms sound the same, the underlying cause and underlying condition is different. Every man with chronic prostatitis is unique in his own self. That is why chronic prostatitis is such an enigma, and that is why it is often very challenging to diagnose and treat.

DEMYSTIFYING PROSTATITIS

That is why many urologists do not know what to do with a prostatitis sufferer (sorry, but it's true). Every man with chronic prostatitis is like a puzzle.

Hence, in order to be successful in healing men with chronic prostatitis, you need to be extremely attentive to every detail of their history, such as health, lifestyle, and sex habits. Once you see a person holistically, you have a much better chance of helping him. But it takes time. You need to spend lots of time listening to their story.

That is why, out of desperation and in an attempt to regulate prostatitis into some kind of system, the honourable group of urologists came up with a classification system. This classification system has been designed to help urologists worldwide as a guide to diagnosis and treatment.

I am going to omit acute prostatitis, since we already mentioned it in the previous chapter. Acute prostatitis is a matter of medical emergency. Chronic prostatitis is a different story.

Basically, chronic prostatitis is divided into Bacterial (NIH category II) and Non-Bacterial (NIH category III). There is also asymptomatic prostatitis (category IV), about which we will talk in a separate chapter[8, 9].

It is here that everything becomes complicated. Let's go back to our old friend John. Assume that on his first visit to his family doctor, the urine culture showed significant infection, especially if it is Escherichia Coli, or other bad types of bacteria (Klebsiella, Pseudomonas aeruginosa, Proteus mirabilis, heavy presence of Enterococcus faecalis, etc.). Bulls eye! We now know it is bacterial prostatitis. Let's treat it with antibiotics and hope for the best.

If you remember, John had a urine test done, which was negative (no infection found), but he was still prescribed an antibiotic, which did not eliminate his symptoms. The Urologist decides to follow the guidelines. He performs a prostate massage and collects urine after it.

DEMYSTIFYING PROSTATITIS

The urine culture test comes back as "no growth," meaning non-bacterial prostatitis. John is sent home with a reassurance that his problem will burn itself out eventually. Hooray!!

But what if the symptoms do not go away?

Unfortunately, nothing is predictable when it comes to chronic prostatitis. Every case is unique. I have personally seen so many men who have taken at least a few courses of antibiotics over the course of a few years, and still presented with signs of chronic prostate infection.

My dear readers, are you sufficiently confused?

How about a statement: "If there is infection detected in a prostate, is the infection causing your symptoms?" That's the Million Dollar Question. If there were ONE correct answer, the person with that answer should surely receive the Nobel Prize in a newly created category: Prostatitis. Even I, with all my many years of experience in this complicated area of specialization, would not dream of being nominated...no one would.

Chronic prostatitis has many causes and complicated factors. Therefore, this classification which divides chronic prostatitis into bacterial and non-bacterial has little to do with real life cases.

Most men develop chronic prostatitis due to an acquired infection. If it's not detected by conventional means, it does not mean it's not there[10, 11, 12].

Once men reach a certain age and especially become sexually active, the prostate is often colonized with microorganisms. Many organisms are shared with other people. The more sexual partners a man has in his lifetime, the more likely he will carry a variety of organisms in his prostate, unless condoms have been used every time he has sex. The good news is this does not mean you are destined to have prostatitis[13, 14].

What are the causes of bacterial prostatitis?

DEMYSTIFYING PROSTATITIS

One of the main causes is that men acquire "hostile" infections through unprotected sexual contact. This is usually the case with younger men who are not in long term relationships.

Another very common scenario occurs when men develop prostatitis caused by their own "domestic" organisms. It usually happens when a man experiences a lot of stress, both physical and emotional, combined with a lack of water intake and excessive alcohol consumption. And here is where the problem begins.

It has been speculated that men can acquire pathogenic bacteria within their own body. Unfortunately, there is extraordinarily little research has been done to back up this theory. Men who suffer from chronic sinus infections, chronic gum or tooth infections, and chronic infections in their gut can have organisms travel via the blood stream into the prostate, and lodge themselves there[15, 16]. My advice, for the sake of your prostate health, is to see your dentist, your ENT (Ear, Nose, Throat) specialist and try to heal these regions as well as possible.

One very legitimate question is, "Why would my own bacteria suddenly turn "nasty" on me?" Many men who are healthy, hard working, married with or without children, or have a partner in life, may ask why it happens to them.

The answer is "because it can". All that is needed is to create a "perfect storm" for it to happen.

During an initial assessment when I see a new patient, I listen to their Prostatitis stories. This is where we pay attention to details and where we do a lot of investigative research.

The patients frequently report important facts: that symptoms often arise during late fall, or early winter; that they have been under a lot of stress lately due to either work or family related issues; that they had to stay at work late at night, drinking lots of coffee or alcohol; that they have had heavy exams, sitting for prolonged hours, being sleep deprived. You can mix and match all these circumstances.

DEMYSTIFYING PROSTATITIS

The bottom line is that they have compromised their natural immune defences due to ongoing stress on their body and... BOOM! Their own bacterial organisms turn "angry", and prostatitis begins.

Moreover, there are men who develop the same problem, under similar circumstances where bacteria are irrelevant. Men suddenly develop a significant muscular spasm around the prostate, which in turn affects prostate physiology, triggers inflammation within the prostate, and once again, prostatitis begins.

There are different types of chronic prostatitis out there. When it comes to bacterial prostatitis, there are some other organisms, which are not bacteria, that can also cause prostatitis. These are organisms such as Mycoplasma Genitalium, Ureaplasma Urealiticum, Trichomonas Vaginalis and Candida Albicans, to name just a few. There are likely other organisms which are guilty of causing prostatitis, about which we are not yet aware.

The organisms I mentioned are not easy to detect, because they are not usually identified by culture. I just want you to be aware of all of the possible causes of prostatitis.

No matter what type of infection may be causing someone's problem, the symptoms for the most part are the same. It is really up to your doctor to try to figure out as much as possible what causes YOUR prostatitis.

In many cases of bacterial prostatitis, there is more than one organism involved. Hence, often, men need to be treated with more than one antibiotic for extended periods of time.

I want to conclude this chapter with a relatively short statement.

What came first, the Chicken or the Egg?

This question amounts to other equally monumental questions such as "To Be or Not to Be?", "Is there life on Mars?", or "How to win a jackpot in the lottery?"

DEMYSTIFYING PROSTATITIS

The "chicken or the egg" question can be asked in a different way: "What started first: the infection or the inflammation?" In many instances it is quite easy to answer. Let's say a man has unprotected sex. A few days later he develops burning on urination, urinary frequency, urgency, pain in the genital area and possibly other unpleasant symptoms. This fellow swears that he has never previously had any of these symptoms. In this case we can say with great confidence that this man most likely acquired an infection, which is responsible for his state of misery. Let's call it a chicken.

On the other hand, let's say our man in question has been living a regular life, goes through periods of high stress as we all do, drinks alcohol sometimes more than average, and spends the bulk of his work day in a seated position. Then, he gradually begins to experience symptoms of pain or discomfort in the genital area, urinary urgency, urinary frequency, and other unpleasant symptoms. In this instance there is no clear evidence that an infection was acquired from an outside source.

Nevertheless, this man responds well to antibiotic treatment. It appears here that lifestyle deviations propelled the onset of symptoms which are inflammatory in nature. Then, an inflammation activated an infection which already existed inside the prostate. Here we have our egg.

My personal opinion is that it does not matter whether the inflammation or the infection came first. Ultimately, we must look after all of them in order to get the patient back on track.

My dear readers: Please take a break, drink some hot water with lemon, or go for a speed walk, and then continue reading.

DEMYSTIFYING PROSTATITIS

CHAPTER 4

What makes men miserable and why?

Many scientific publications have thoroughly documented as dismal the quality of life of men suffering from chronic prostatitis (CP). It has been compared to such debilitating conditions as diabetes, heart attack, angina, congestive heart failure and Crohn's Disease. In other words, CP is often compared to life threatening conditions in terms of how men feel physically, emotionally, and psychologically[17, 18, 19].

Why?

Chronic prostatitis, though an "annoying condition" which presents itself with a variety of symptoms, is by no means a serious threat to your overall health. Let me say that again: it is by no means a serious threat to your overall health. Nevertheless, it has a dramatic impact on one's quality of life, sense of well-being and emotional state. The same scientific publications indicated that the severity of the symptoms, especially pain, have a huge impact on quality of life. There are also socioeconomic factors involved. Men with less education and lower income tend to suffer a greater impact on their quality of life[20, 21, 22].

Another significant covariant applies to men with illness-oriented behaviour rather than wellness-oriented behaviour. Men with the former behavioral pattern also tend to experience a worse quality of life.

Let me present one of my patients as an example:

John is 42 years old and works as an IT analyst. He comes to my clinic for an initial assessment complaining about constant aching pains in the perineal area, groin, tip of the penis and lower back. He reports a "golf ball" pain in the perineum (area between scrotum and

DEMYSTIFYING PROSTATITIS

anus) while sitting, burning pain after ejaculation, difficulty maintaining erections, reduced sense of climax and low libido. He also reports urinary urgency and frequency, needing to get out of bed to urinate up to three times a night. John feels depressed and anxious. He has no motivation to do his job or engage in any family activities with his wife and children. John tells me that his symptoms started about two years ago and despite a few courses of antibiotics, his symptoms are only getting worse. He has seen his family doctor many times. He has also seen at least two different urologists. Ultimately, they all gave up on him. He was told that he has non-bacterial Chronic Prostatitis/Chronic Pain Syndrome (CP/CPPS) and there is nothing much else they can do for him. Their last advice to him was to get used to this condition and hope that one day it would go away on its own.

While John is telling me his story, he constantly checks his notes. He wants to be as specific as possible. He wants to describe all his symptoms in every minute detail. He looks pale, jittery, has a hard time sitting still. He tells me that he has not had a normal night's sleep in months. At the end of his story, John starts to cry.

My dear readers, believe me: it is heartbreaking to watch an adult man cry in my office.

Please remember, he does not cry because he has just learned about a terminal disease which will shorten his life by many years. He cries because he is depressed, has constant pain, hasn't slept well in months, doesn't know what is truly wrong with him and no one will help him.

Of course, the name John is fictional, but the story is real. I have seen many men with very similar accounts. Some men even confess later on, after they got better, that they contemplated suicide.

How is it possible that such a small gland, which holds a very limited value in a man's physiology, can inflict so much suffering comparable to the most debilitating diseases?

And the answer is: we do not know.

I am personally not aware of a single scientific study which states that men with CP/CPPS suffer a very poor quality of life due to only one single cause. And this is why there is very little scientific research on prostatitis: because typically there is no single cause. It is usually multifactorial. This is the most truthful statement we can come up with. There are many factors which can affect a man's quality of life.

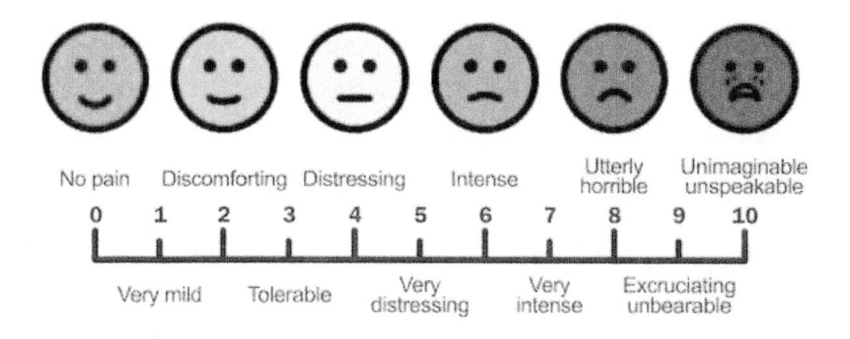

Intensity of pain is definitely a factor. If someone has pain at level 7-10 on the Visual Analog Scale (a validated, subjective tool for measuring acute and chronic pain), and this degree of pain endures for a long time, it is not surprising that this will affect his quality of life.

Effective pain control becomes a paramount concern. I have seen many men who had to take opioid drugs for pain control. It is far from an ideal situation, but it may be a necessary evil.

Fortunately, now we have many options instead of prescribing painkillers such as opioids, which can provide pain control without inflicting significant side effects or risking addiction. Please remember that this book is not a textbook designed for health professionals as a guide on CP/CPPS. Therefore, I am not going to list the names of drugs which would be recommended to treat chronic pelvic pain. Many urologists, pain specialists and general practitioners are well informed about these drugs. Obviously, every patient is a unique case and, therefore, treatment choices should be very specific to his case. The best approach to finding the right treatment method would be to determine the principal cause of pain first and then act accordingly.

Level of Education and Income:

Scientific data indicates that men with a lower level of education and low income suffer a poorer quality of life than men with a higher education (College or University graduates) and higher income (over $50,000/year).

First of all, most of the data collected for this study (21) occurred in the United States. When it comes to income level, I am certain that men who live in communities with limited access to health care will have greater difficulty getting diagnosed and treated. As a note to my Canadian readers, the statistics on Canadian rates are almost non-existent[18].

When it comes to education, I believe this factor has a significant impact on quality of life in men with CP/CPPS. In the era of the internet, almost everything is researchable and can be accessed by anyone assuming they have access to a computer or cell phone with internet capabilities, which not everyone does. My interpretation of education, in this case, is what men read on the internet about prostatitis and how they interpret what they read. Many men just read about symptoms they develop over time. With this knowledge they go see their family doctor, present the case and let the health care provider do the rest.

Another type of patients, especially those who have been to many doctors unsuccessfully, read everything they can find on the subject of prostatitis. They overwhelm themselves with too much information. Many of them read scientific research publications and try to apply the information acquired to their own condition. I understand that they do it out of desperation. They are not doctors, moreover urologists.

DEMYSTIFYING PROSTATITIS

They do not know how to filter all this information. Many of them become fixated on some idea, which, in reality, has no relevance to their problem. As a result, there is more anxiety and dissatisfaction with the health care they receive[22, 23].

There are many other men, especially younger men, who actively participate in chat groups with men who suffer from similar conditions all over the world. They exchange their disease history, symptoms and treatments. This is also often one of the worst-case scenarios.

They try to apply treatment advice given by some stranger and usually get nothing good out of it. They become even more fixated and frustrated. They keep going back to these chat groups. They keep talking to other men who tell them that this condition is for life, and there is nothing that can be done about it. Now, they are not only frustrated, but completely miserable. Many withdraw from social life, stop exercising, limit communication with family and friends. What makes it even worse is that they become addicted to the internet, especially chat groups. Subsequently these men end up having a dismal quality of life. In summary, men suffering from CP/CPPS have a much worse quality of life when they are illness-oriented.

Scientific studies[24] report that men who are wellness-oriented experience a much better quality of life. And that is actually very true. When I talk to my patients, I know exactly who is illness-oriented and who is not. If my patient looks grim, anxious, shares with me many stories he reads on the internet, and has been to more than two doctors in the past, I know that he is illness-oriented. And I know that I need to do a lot of intervention by means of counseling and education.

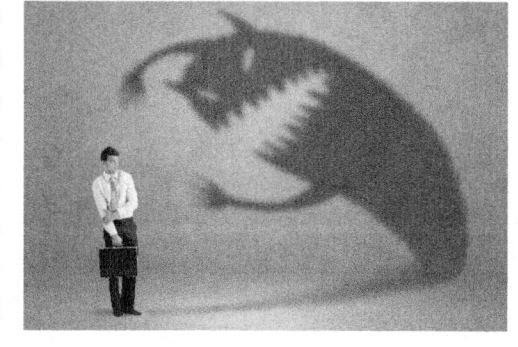

DEMYSTIFYING PROSTATITIS

I believe that one of the main reasons why many men suffer poor quality of life when they have CP/CPPS is fear of the unknown. They do not know exactly what is going on with them because doctors often are not able to establish a correct diagnosis. They often develop even more anxiety and fear when the treatment they receive does not help. Their thoughts start racing in different directions. They start reading too many websites, or even worse, go on forums where shared information can be very questionable and misleading.

And, here you go, illness-oriented poor quality of life in its bloom.

What kind of conclusions can we draw from everything discussed above?

First of all, reassurance and knowledge are key factors in making men less stressed, less anxious and, therefore, in improving their quality of life.

Most men who come to our clinic experience significant anxiety, stress and poor quality of life due to not knowing what exactly is happening with them. That is even more true for men who have been to a few doctors and have never received a full understanding about their condition.

Fear of the unknown seems to be one of the very significant factors in causing poor quality of life. That is where our responsibility comes as health professionals in educating our patients about this condition to the best of our knowledge. It would also be advisable that men suffering from CP/CPPS try to educate themselves through reputable sources of information. This is a principal reason why I have written this book.

Second, once men are empowered with the knowledge about their condition, they need to develop a strategy of how to deal with it. An appropriate mindset is very important here. Men need to keep all lines of communication open. It's very important that they do not become introverts and keep everything to themselves, which would be more likely to cause increased anxiety and depression.

It is obvious that finding a health provider who can help to establish a correct diagnosis, educate the man about his condition, and put forward a treatment plan, is vitally important.

But it is also very important that a man suffering with CP/CPPS communicates well with his loved ones, whether it is a spouse, partner or anyone else close to him. Being able to openly discuss his problem with someone would help to relieve anxiety and establish a supportive environment conducive to healing.

We are very well aware of support groups for people suffering from different types of cancers. They are doing great work in helping people with cancer in terms of emotional and practical support. Unfortunately, I do not think sufferers from CP/CPPS receive the same level of support. There are some websites and forums on this subject, but it is not clear whether any are moderated by or receive input from a medical professional who can help correct the sharing of misinformation. Therefore, building support from family and friends would help to establish positive reinforcement and provide an optimistic outlook toward healing.

Third, it is important to establish wellness-oriented behaviour rather than illness-oriented behaviour.

As I mentioned previously it is so common that men with CP/CPPS often withdraw from their normal life activities. They stop exercising because they feel no motivation, or they are too lethargic to do it. They do not want to socialize with other people like they used to. They spend too much time on the internet reading everything they can find about their condition. They do not share their fears and issues with their loved ones. There are men who begin to underperform on

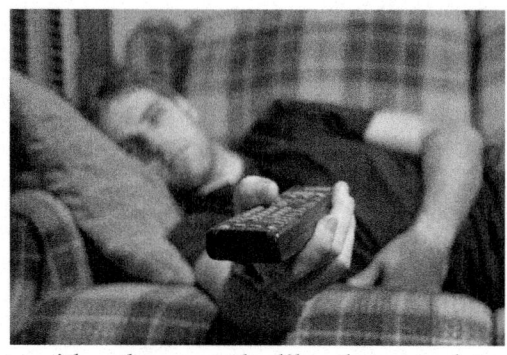

DEMYSTIFYING PROSTATITIS

their jobs. Some of them become debilitated to such a degree that they are forced to go on short-term, or sometimes, long-term disability and I have met and dealt with men who have done just that due to CP/CPPS.

They usually suffer from the most severe forms of this condition, complicated by a significant impact on their psychological and emotional state. These men require as much help as they can get. There is no single person who can solve all their problems. They need a multidisciplinary approach to their treatment, such as a Primary Care Physician, Urologist, Psychologist, Physiotherapist, Pain Specialist, and possibly other auxiliary health providers such as an acupuncturist, naturopathic specialist, or dietician.

You can ask me a legitimate question. What can I do myself to help in dealing with this condition? The answer is "Live a wellness-oriented lifestyle". What does this mean? It means that you need to divert and focus your attention on mental and physical health. Utilize all means possible to deal with fear, anxiety and depression by educating yourself by searching out and reading well-validated sources of medical information such as university or medical center websites, seeking reassurance, staying positive and keeping all lines of communication open.

If you feel that your emotional state is not in good control, seek professional help by consulting with a Psychologist, or Primary Care Physician. There are many other means that can be effective in helping you to stay wellness-oriented, such as meditation, self-relaxation techniques, yoga (Raja, Hatha Yoga, etc.), Reflexology, or a nice vacation somewhere warm and sunny.

By the way, there are many men with CP/CPPS who report that they feel very well while on vacation. Do you know why? The answer is simple: They get away from their daily routine, they do not sit all day long by the computers or steering wheels (hello truck drivers!), they swim, sunbathe, and do lots of walking. Basically, they do everything they need to counteract their prostate inflammation and pelvic muscle spasm.

Oh wait, I think we may have just found the ultimate solution to treating CP/CPPS: Wouldn't it be great if all men with CP could go for one long never-ending vacation? Yes, it would, but, unfortunately, we live in reality, not virtual reality. But, why not give it a try? Even if you live in a climate that has cold, gloomy weather for almost 6 months of the year, please try to go out somewhere as often as you can. Try doing things you enjoy most, but with some exceptions.

If it's a form of exercise, please try to keep to it with regularity. However, avoid spinning classes, or bicycling in general, unless you have a special seat, which eliminates pressure behind your testicles (perineum). Any hard pressure in this area can lead to more pain due to activation of prostate inflammation and muscle spasm around the prostate.

If you have a desk job, try to get up from your chair at least every 20-30 minutes and go for a quick walk somewhere for 1-2 minutes. Just pretend that you are doing something important and your supervisor will be pleased, unless of course you are the supervisor yourself, in which case you won't need permission.

There is another group of men who do not necessarily work at a desk but suffer from CP/CPPS. These are men who sit long hours at the steering wheel: truck drivers (especially long-haul drivers), taxi drivers, tractor operators and operators of other machinery who are forced to sit for hours on seats that are often quite hard. Some of the less fortunate ones do not have good shock absorbers, which makes symptoms even worse. Unfortunately, you cannot advise individuals with such jobs to get up and go for a walk every 30 minutes as they would never get their work done. What other options do they have to alleviate pain while sitting in their trucks, cars, tractors and rocket ships?

DEMYSTIFYING PROSTATITIS

The answer is cushions. There is no one single type of cushion that will fit everyone. Some men use donut shaped cushions. Other men use horseshoe shaped cushions. Some feel better on softer cushions. For others it makes symptoms worse. It is a matter of trial and error. The general idea is to minimize pressure from the seat towards the perineal area (saddle area) and, therefore, reduce the ill effect on the perineal muscles and the prostate.

Also, pay attention to the temperature of your seat, especially if you have a leather type seat. In the winter, when you get into your car, the seat is very cold, unless your vehicle is always inside a garage. A cold seat will immediately cause a spasm of the pelvic floor muscles and will activate inflammation in the prostate, causing more symptoms. I usually recommend a simple trick to help overcome this unnecessary trigger: a piece of sheepskin. Just keep it on the top of your car seat. It will keep it warm. It is a natural wool which is breathable. That means less water condensation on the skin of your perineal area. Therefore, it is good for your prostate and surrounding muscles.

Overall, avoid sitting on cold surface for the same reason. Avoid exposure to cold especially below your waist. Therefore, if you live in a place with a cold winter, wear a jacket which covers your behind.

Remember to keep your feet warm and dry as well. Prostate likes dry and warm environment. There are many men who develop a bad flare up of prostatitis after freezing their "behind" or their feet.

Another word of wisdom for you: If you feel that your bladder is full, do not hold it back. Make sure that you go for a pee whatever place you can. I wonder if there are fewer men suffering from prostatitis in France. I have personally seen and smelled many instances of men peeing on a wall or a fence. I think that we are blessed in Canada, or maybe in the entirety of North America, with way more access to public washrooms where men can pee under more civilized and sanitary conditions. I have seen quite a few young men

DEMYSTIFYING PROSTATITIS

who develop prostatitis just because they were holed up in a car with a very full bladder. This risk factor is even more relevant to older men with Enlarged Prostate (BPH). Almost every man with BPH report a significant decrease in a force of urination when their bladder is very full. In case of BPH this situation puts men on the edge of tipping point. They are running into a risk of a complete blockage (Acute Urinary retention). That is a medical emergency, which requires a catheter insertion into a bladder to relieve obstruction. So, the take home message here is: If you feel a strong desire to pee, go for it. Let it out and thank a higher power for letting it happen.

Now, a suggestion of regular exercise applies to every man whether you are a desk work person or a driver.

If you do not want to go to the gym or are too busy, exercise at home. Try to do stretching exercises for muscles in the pelvic area as often as you can. If you are not sure what and how to do them, consult a physiotherapist. Stretching muscles in the pelvic area helps to relieve congestion, boosts blood flow and, therefore, assists in healing.

If you master good yoga skills, meditation, and self-relaxation techniques, try to practice them on a regular basis. They are great tools toward boosting the healing process. And of course, don't forget about the application of heat. Most men with CP/CPPS experience relief from their symptoms by applying heat. Whether it is a hot sitz bath or a heating pad, do not hesitate to use them. It is clear that these measures are for symptom relief, but if they help to feel better why not use them? Heat helps to increase blood flow to the pelvic area, both the prostate and pelvic muscles. It helps to relax muscles around the prostate. If you find heat helpful, please use it whenever it feels necessary.

We have talked here about wellness-oriented behaviour, which is definitely not complete. A big part of wellness-oriented behaviour is your dietary habits, as they can play an important role in either

DEMYSTIFYING PROSTATITIS

supporting CP/CPPS or combating it. For this reason, I decided to dedicate a single chapter specifically to diet, which you'll find later in this book.

Please take a break, go for a quick walk, conquer the world and then keep reading. We will see you soon!

CHAPTER 5

That time you have problems in the bedroom, and it isn't the snoring

My dear readers, as you can see, this chapter is dedicated to the most intimate part of our lives: life in the bedroom. These problems aren't related to snoring or insomnia. They're about sex and all problems related to it.

There are a significant number of men who suffer from Chronic Prostatitis/Chronic Pain Syndrome (CP/CPPS), which may be accompanied by various forms of sexual dysfunction. Allow me to remind you what the most common symptoms of sexual dysfunction are:

- Difficulty to attain and maintain an erection
- Premature or delayed ejaculation
- Low sexual drive (low libido)
- Pain during or shortly after ejaculation
- Reduced sensation of orgasm (climax)
- Presence of blood in semen (hematospermia)

Men with CP/CPPS do not necessarily experience all the symptoms listed above. In fact, some men with CP/CPPS have no sexual dysfunction issues at all.

The scientific data on this subject is very limited. Nevertheless, from scientific publications available to us, we know that 30% to 50% of men with CP/CPPS present signs and symptoms of erectile dysfunction. It has been reported that up to 50% of men with CP/CPPS report pain with ejaculation. We also know that most men who experience some form of sexual dysfunction score higher on the psychological domain and symptoms severity. In other words, men

DEMYSTIFYING PROSTATITIS

who experience signs of depression, anxiety and/or have more severe symptoms of CP/CPPS are most likely to suffer from ED (Erectile Dysfunction). This is true for men of all ages from 18 to 65.

Let's take a look at one of my patient's cases. For privacy's sake, we will call him Michael.

Michael is 42 years old, married, with two children. He developed symptoms of prostatitis eighteen months ago (pain in the genital area, perineal pain, burning during urination) and has been on a few antibiotics without substantial resolution of his symptoms. Three months later, he developed difficulty maintaining his erection and developed pain with ejaculation, low sex drive and a decreased sense of climax. During an assessment, Michael reported that he felt very anxious and depressed due to ongoing issues with his prostate and sexual dysfunction. He was able to perform sexual intercourse with his partner, but it became more of a burden than a pleasure. Michael reported that his relationship with his partner started to deteriorate and as a result, he is more irritable, unhappy and tries to avoid any kind of sexual contact with his partner unless he is really pressured into it.

This is a classic example of a man suffering from CP/CPPS. It is important to note that men with sexual dysfunction develop it after an onset of CP/CPPS. This means that the successful treatment of CP/CPPS will help to restore their sexual function to its normal state. I want to emphasize to those of you who suffer from CP/CPPS and sexual dysfunction - do not despair. If you developed sexual problems along with CP/CPPS, this will be a temporary problem. The more your CP/CPPS is under control or the closer you are to being cured, the more likely you will recover from sexual dysfunction.

Now let us get more specific about the various types of sexual dysfunction.

Erectile dysfunction

One significant presentation is difficulty with obtaining and/or maintaining an erection during sexual activity. Many men with

DEMYSTIFYING PROSTATITIS

CP/CPPS report a loss of spontaneous erections. These are erections which have nothing to do with sexual arousal. They occur overnight or upon waking in the morning. Some men with CP/CPPS who are still able to preserve erections during sexual activity seem to be quite troubled by the loss of spontaneous erections. You can only imagine how men with ED feel. There is no doubt that the psychological impact is very significant: these men feel less confident in themselves, they lose their sense of masculinity, and develop significant anxiety and depression. They think that there is something seriously wrong with them and that they have become impotent for life. Once men get themselves into this state of mind, it only makes matters worse. They are likely to experience more severe symptoms of CP/CPPS and ED. When a man develops ED, he is less inclined to engage in sexual activity, which therefore diminishes the frequency of sexual activity, and increases the sexual dissatisfaction for both partners. The relationship's discord only grows from here.

I have now painted a not-so-pretty picture. Unfortunately, this is the reality for many men who suffer from CP/CPPS. To this day, we do not know what causes erectile dysfunction in men with CP/CPPS. We only know that it is more likely to happen in men who have more severe symptoms of pain and men who suffer a psychological impact (anxiety, emotional stress, depression).

My advice, especially to younger men with CP/CPPS and who suffer with ED, is to take good care of your prostate and pelvic muscles. As a rule, there is nothing wrong with you anatomically. If you have had all basic examinations done which have ruled out significant structural problems, your sexual function will return once you get your CP/CPPS under control. Utilize all necessary means (i.e. meditation, self-relaxation techniques, yoga, reflexology, psychotherapy) to get your anxiety and depression under control. If you need medication to help you achieve better control, so be it. If you were a completely healthy person who never suffered from severe

DEMYSTIFYING PROSTATITIS

anxiety and/or depression prior to developing CP/CPPS, you will be alright. Your sex life will return to normal.

Here is my message to your partners - and my message is the same regardless of whether your partner is male or female. If your partner suffers from CP/CPPS and as a result, has developed ED, please do not take it personally. It is not because of you. You are as desirable a partner to them now as you were before. Please be patient and stay calm and relaxed. Encourage your partner to open up to you and share all of his fears and concerns. Men who suffer with CP/CPPS, especially if they have ED as well, need someone to talk to. Who is a better person to be open to, as it relates to their sex life, than their sexual partner? If you care about each other and are passionate about each other, you should find a way to talk openly without judgment or embarrassment. Try to communicate any sexual concerns you both experience and come to a mutual agreement on how and what type of sexual intimacy you want to maintain in order to keep your partner relaxed, calm and reassured. It will become a powerful tool in helping men with ED and CP/CPPS find the road to a full recovery.

Premature ejaculation

Premature ejaculation (PE), which is another common sexual dysfunction that happens to men with CP, is when a man ejaculates sooner than he or his partner desires. This, of course, begs the question: if a man lasts one hour during sex but his partner is still dissatisfied, does it mean that this man suffers from PE? I would suggest not. Therefore, we have developed a clinical definition of PE. Men have PE if they ejaculate within a maximum of 3 minutes into sexual activity, whether it is sexual intercourse or masturbation. Psychological distress could also be a factor in PE as well.

In clinical practice we recognize two types of premature ejaculation: Primary and Secondary.

Primary PE is defined as a condition man have always experienced since the onset of their sex life.

DEMYSTIFYING PROSTATITIS

Secondary (i.e., acquired) PE means that men develop it later in life. There are other reasons why men develop secondary PE: relationship issues, anxiety, erectile dysfunction, neurological conditions, diabetes, to name a few. Since our book focuses on prostatitis, we are not going to discuss PE caused by factors other than chronic prostatitis.

The overall prevalence of PE is very high. It has been estimated that 1-in-3 men worldwide have experienced PE at least once in their lifetime. Severe PE can definitely become a source of emotional distress for both partners. It is especially significant for younger men who are single and trying to establish a long-term relationship. A few methods on treating PE include desensitization techniques, behavioral therapy, and medications.

When PE happens to men with CP, it is usually the most pronounced during a flare up of prostatitis. We do not know why men with CP develop PE. My personal opinion is that an inflamed prostate also triggers inflammation of neural receptors (neural endings) located within the prostate gland itself. As a result, there is a lower threshold of sexual stimuli, especially one directed towards the penile area. Therefore, premature ejaculation takes place.

The good news here is that once inflammation in the prostate subsides (regardless of whether it is bacterial or not), men recover their usual ejaculatory reflex.

The underlying message here is that men who develop PE due to CP need to treat their prostatitis by whatever means determined by their health providers to solve their PE problem. Nevertheless, if their premature ejaculation problems persist, they need to consult their doctor and look into other possible causes. After all, any type of PE which is not related to prostatitis will be addressed with a similar approach as we mentioned earlier in our chapter.

DEMYSTIFYING PROSTATITIS

Delayed ejaculation

Delayed ejaculation is not a common problem in men with Chronic Prostatitis, but it has been reported. Delayed ejaculation means that for a man to reach his climax (orgasm), it takes much longer than he desires. Medical science poorly understands this phenomenon in the context of chronic prostatitis. We observe this mostly in older men who are in their 60's and above.

It is our understanding that this problem is linked to the peripheral nervous system. The neural endings located in the skin of the penis, particularly in the head of the penis, suffer some degenerative changes. As a result, these neural endings require much more stimulation and more local stimulation to trigger the complex chain of physiological reactions which lead to climax. I have encountered a few men in their 70's who complained about an inability to achieve climax during sexual intercourse. Nevertheless, they could achieve it through masturbation.

If this problem occurs due to a flare up of prostatitis, it will be resolved once symptoms of prostatitis subside. If, however, delayed ejaculation occurs due to peripheral nerve degeneration, it is there to stay. There is no medicine which can specifically address this issue, and only adjustments in sexual practices can help amend this problem. Both partners need to know that men with delayed ejaculation require more direct stimulation especially toward the head of the penis to trigger a more timely orgasm. The good news is, this problem seldom becomes a troublesome point between partners, unlike erectile dysfunction and premature ejaculation.

Reduced sensation of climax

A reduced sensation of climax is a very common complaint among men with active symptoms of prostatitis. They often report that climax is not as strong as before and that when ejaculation takes place, the seminal fluid leaks out rather than shoots out as it normally does. These symptoms are usually caused by inflammation in the prostate, but they can also be caused by increased spasticity of the muscles located in close proximity to the prostate and seminal vesicles. In order to address this problem, the prostate inflammation needs to be treated. Whether it is caused by an infection or not is a subject to address with your physician. If a problem with weak ejaculation continues to persist in the absence of symptoms of active prostatitis, pelvic floor muscles require assessment and specialized management if appropriate, which is usually administered by pelvic floor physiotherapists.

There is a whole range of special exercises and other techniques being implemented to treat pelvic floor muscle dysfunction. I have seen many men with chronic pelvic pain, a reduced force of ejaculation and other symptoms who have benefited from pelvic floor muscle rehabilitation programs, only after their prostatitis condition has improved to the level of full remission.

Pain during or after ejaculation

This is another very common symptom in men with CP/CPPS and it has been estimated that at least half of men with CP/CPPS suffer from pain during or after ejaculation. The intensity of pain may vary from just a slight discomfort to excruciating pain, which makes men scream vocally or internally. The location of pain may vary but many men feel pain along the penile shaft, often pointing out that the glans penis (i.e., the head of the penis) hurts the most. Other men experience pain in the testicles, perineal area, low back and groin. Nonetheless, the location of pain varies from person to person. Many men report pain in just one area while other men report pain in a few different locations. The type of pain can also vary. Some men report a dull, throbbing pain while other men report a burning pain. As I mentioned earlier, approximately half of men with CP experience pain during or right after ejaculation. The intensity of pain definitely has an impact on men's sexual behaviour. The more severe the pain, the more likely men will develop erectile dysfunction or premature ejaculation, and as a result, withdrawal from sexual activity

DEMYSTIFYING PROSTATITIS

altogether. The latter point carries very serious consequences. A man with significant pain related to ejaculation loses interest in sex. Logically, who would want to engage in sex if it hurts?

Let's look at an example:

John, a 42 year old engineer, married with two children, comes to our clinic for an initial assessment with his wife by his side. (As a side note, when a partner accompanies the patient, this is usually a very good sign. It usually means the partner is engaged in the patient's problem and that there is an open line of communication). John reports symptoms of prostatitis such as pain in various pelvic areas, urinary frequency, urgency, and some burning during urination. He also reports having significant pain in his perineal area during and right after ejaculation which lasts for hours. John was diagnosed with CP/CPPS about three years ago. He has been having ejaculatory pain for the last two years. When we discuss his intimate life in detail, John admits that the last time he had sex with his wife was about 12 months ago. He admits that he still ejaculates by masturbation every 2-3 weeks. He does it not due to a sexual urge, but because he read online that he needs to ejaculate to help his prostatitis problem. John looks visibly distressed, his voice trembles on occasion and his body language conveys heightened anxiety. The good news here is that his wife is sitting by his side holding his hand.

I am intentionally emphasizing the presence of his wife as good news, despite the overall severity of John's condition. I have seen many men who complained of exactly the same symptoms, withdrew from sex for many months, but presented alone. They too have long term partners, with whom they often do not have open communication. There are different reasons for this, but the end result is the same. These men suffer alone, in silence. Their stress level, anxiety and depression are ten times worse than John's. Their partners typically take it personally and the relationship develops a rift. Therefore, the problems build on the horizon and it doesn't get any easier.

DEMYSTIFYING PROSTATITIS

I am afraid that I have painted quite a gloomy picture here. Unfortunately, it is a reality which many men with CP face on a daily basis. But there is a silver lining here. The overwhelming majority of men who have pain with ejaculation will have this pain disappear or drastically diminish upon comprehensive prostatitis treatment. Ejaculatory pain has no specific cause. It is almost always the result of significant prostate inflammation regardless of whether it is infectious or non-infectious in origin. It can also be caused by inflamed, hypertonic pelvic floor muscles and/or inflamed neural endings within both the prostate and the muscles.

In many men it is all of the above. Hence, again, we need to take a multidisciplinary approach to the severe cases. The comprehensive treatment of infection, inflammation and pelvic floor muscle rehabilitation are ultimate solutions to resolving this debilitating disorder. Reducing and eliminating pain with ejaculation not only makes men who suffer feel better, but it also saves relationships, strengthens intimate bonds and restores mental health.

Decreased sex drive (libido)

It is not uncommon for men to report a decrease in sex drive during a flare up of symptoms. Low sex drive is a common complaint in men over the age of 45. The older the men, the higher the incidence of low sex drive. It is a physiological phenomenon of declining levels of testosterone (male sex hormone) in aging men. When men in the age group of 40 to 65 complain about low sex drive, doctors often search for the cause. There are many causes for men to report low sex drive at a younger age. Very often it has nothing to do with hormones. When men experience symptoms of active prostatitis, their sex drive will diminish simply because they do not feel well. It is logical that if you are in pain, that sexual activity is not your priority.

As we mentioned earlier, at least half of men with prostatitis experience pain during or after ejaculation. Consequently, the whole sexual experience becomes much less pleasurable and men's desire for sex diminishes. In turn, they engage in sex much less often than

DEMYSTIFYING PROSTATITIS

they would otherwise. Some men, during a flare up of prostatitis, try to have sex with their partners with the same regularity as during a "healthy" period. They do it despite the pain and in this case, they feel that it is their obligation to keep their partners sexually satisfied. Unfortunately, such sexual behaviour often causes more sexual dissatisfaction for men as it adds more stress and anxiety, and only worsens prostatitis symptoms. On the other hand, when men withdraw from sex, sometimes for a long time (i.e., weeks or months), this can put a lot of strain on their spousal relationships and can significantly disrupt family dynamics.

The most important strategy to deal with this situation is to discuss all these issues and concerns with your partner. It is very important to let your partner know exactly what and how you feel. Explain to your partner exactly what you experience and the reasons why sex is not appealing to you at the moment. We can only hope that your partner will understand and provide maximum support. The good news is, once symptoms of prostatitis subside, sexual desire goes back to normal and life goes on as before.

There are many other reasons that men may report a low sex drive. Many men with chronic prostatitis, even when they are not symptomatic, still complain about it. Typically, these men belong to a middle-aged group, are married with children, and keep high stress jobs. In some cases, when a blood test is administered for hormonal panels (male hormones), we find hormonal deficiency. These men as a rule will require hormonal replacement therapy (TRT), or some other treatment to boost their testosterone levels, which in turn will improve their libido. Nevertheless, most men who complain about low sex drive usually have normal levels of testosterone. Further, there are many other reasons for low sex drive that are either health-related or simply due to a certain lifestyle. I am not going to delve into health-related reasons since it is a separate subject demanding a significant medical deep-dive. This is something that should be discussed with your primary physician and dealt with accordingly.

DEMYSTIFYING PROSTATITIS

Most men from the age of 35 to 60 complain about low libido due to lifestyle issues. There are many factors which can cause these issues such as diet, stress, sedentary lifestyle, chronic sleep deprivation, relationship breakdown, and the routine of daily life.

I often challenge a patient who complaints about low sex drive but is otherwise a very healthy individual in a loving steady relationship, to go on a nice long vacation of at least one week - and definitely without the kids. Surprise, surprise! Most of them report that their sex life during their vacation was way better than when they are living with their daily routines.

We all know the moral of this story. Try to keep your life as active as possible. Eat healthy, do not be a couch potato, try to break a routine as often as you can by going places and you will do much better. Interestingly enough, the same advice applies to men with chronic prostatitis. I would go even further by saying this applies to men with chronic prostatitis even more than men who do not have it.

Blood in Semen (Hematospermia)

It is a very traumatic experience for men to see blood in their semen. The good news is that hematospermia is very rare as it is due to a serious disease, such as cancer.

There is very limited research available on the prevalence of hematospermia and its causes. It has been suggested that at least 15% of men with hematospermia develop it without any obvious reason. We call it idiopathic hematospermia. It happens on one or more occasions and then disappears for good. Usually men with idiopathic (unknown cause) hematospermia do not have any other symptoms. The most common cause of hematospermia is infectious-inflammatory condition in the urogenital tract. Men with acute epididymitis (acute infection of the testicular epididymis, the convoluted duct behind the testis, along which sperm passes to the vas deferens) often observe blood in the semen. It is also common for

DEMYSTIFYING PROSTATITIS

men with an acute phase of chronic prostatitis to report blood in their semen.

I usually ask my patients about the colour or shade of blood they see in their semen. If they report bright red blood in their semen it is usually due to active inflammation of the prostate, especially in areas close to the ejaculatory ducts and urethra. When men report a rusty/dark brownish colour, it usually means the issue has originated from the seminal vesicles. Hence, it also means that along with prostatitis they also might suffer from vesiculitis (inflammation of seminal vesicles). Men who have prostatitis along with hematospermia often present with other symptoms typical of prostatitis. In most cases, hematospermia is caused by an infection located in both the prostate and seminal vesicles. The majority of men with hematospermia and prostatitis/vesiculitis can be cured from hematospermia after appropriate treatment with antibiotics.

Unfortunately, there are rare cases where men continue to report blood in their semen despite the most comprehensive treatment. We have had these men tested with pelvic MRI (Magnetic Resonance Imaging), which showed the presence of blood clots in one or both seminal vesicles. It is also worth mentioning that if men report blood in their semen, even with the presence of prostatitis, a note should be taken whether any blood thinning medication has been taken. Inflammatory erosion of tissue in the prostate or seminal vesicle can cause small blood leakage. But if blood thinning medication is being taken, it will make the small bleeding much more prolonged.

The bottom line is that hematospermia is not a serious or life-threatening condition. It causes a much stronger psychological and emotional impact on both men who suffer from this condition and their partners, rather than the impact itself on men's health. For example, hematospermia is listed as one of the symptoms of prostate cancer. That is one of the reasons why many men are highly disturbed by its presence. If that is the case, it usually occurs in men with a very locally advanced disease. In developed countries where screening for

DEMYSTIFYING PROSTATITIS

prostate cancer has become a regular part of public health care, diagnosing men in late stages of prostate cancer has become much less common. Also, most men who develop prostate cancer as an actual disease are in their 60s' or older. The older men are, the more likely they will be diagnosed with some type of prostate cancer. Most men who present with hematospermia are younger and have an active sex life, therefore making it much less likely that prostrate cancer is the cause of their hematospermia.

My take home message with regards to hematospermia is not to panic. Address this issue with your doctor, make sure that your prostate and seminal vesicles are being checked for infection and inflammation. If you are at an appropriate age, screening for prostate cancer should be performed on a regular basis and if any issues arise they should be dealt with in a timely manner with the help of your health care providers.

Life goes on and so does this book. Please take a break and then move on to the next chapter.

DEMYSTIFYING PROSTATITIS

CHAPTER 6

To Ejaculate or Not to Ejaculate, that is the question!

The reason for this close scrutiny of the topic of sexual function and sexual problems related to chronic prostatitis is that a man's sexual activity has a direct impact on whether he will develop CP in the first place, and because men with CP frequently experience sexual problems. In this chapter, I will focus more specifically on ejaculation. In my personal experience in treating men who suffer from CP/CPPS, I find that an overwhelming majority of my patients report some degree of ejaculatory problems, at least at some point in the course of the disease. We have mentioned these symptoms in the previous chapters, but they bear repeating:

- Pain or burning in the genital area during or after ejaculation
- Weak force of ejaculation (seminal fluid leaks out rather than ejects by propulsion/squirts)
- Reduced sensation of climax (orgasm), no sense of pleasure
- Flare of symptoms of CP/CPPS after ejaculation (pain, burning on urination, urinary urgency, frequency, fatigue)
- Reduction in symptoms of CP (sense of pressure, discomfort in genital area, heavy sensation) after ejaculation

Overall, it is clear that ejaculation plays an important role in the quality of life of men who suffer from CP/CPPS.

Usually ejaculation is achieved by the act of sexual activity, such as sexual intercourse or masturbation.

There is a separate entity, such as nocturnal ejaculation ("wet dreams"), that play a part of men's sexual development and this usually occurs post puberty when men become sexually mature.

DEMYSTIFYING PROSTATITIS

Sometimes men in their 20s' and 30s' report "wet dreams". Often, this occurs when men abstain for a long time from any type of sexual activity that would lead to ejaculation.

The majority of men, especially in a younger age group (16 - 50 years old), experience regular ejaculations, either through sexual intercourse and/or masturbation. To healthy men without prostatitis, I say "go for it". It does not matter how often or in what kind of sexual activity you engage. If you feel well, do whatever you want and as often you want.

It is a different matter when we deal with someone suffering from prostatitis. The most frequently asked question I get from my patients is "How often should I ejaculate?"

During an initial assessment with a new patient, this question comes up very often when we touch on the subject of ejaculation. Most men with CP research their condition on the internet and the majority of them have already been seen and treated by their family doctor and/or other GPs and Urologists. Men often inquire about the frequency of ejaculation and they frequently receive the same answer, whether it is from the internet or from their doctor: "Try to ejaculate as often as possible, because it will help to reduce symptoms of prostatitis."

When I am asked this question, I can not give them such a generic response. The right answer is: "it depends". There is never a universal or "generic" solution to any one problem encountered by men with prostatitis. Prostatitis is a multifaceted condition that does not lend itself to a "one size fits all" approach.

I have seen many men who complained about the worsening of their pain and urinary symptoms after ejaculation. Some of them continued to practice regular ejaculations up to 4-5 times per week despite suffering these symptoms. They simply continued doing so because either somebody told them, or they read on the internet that frequent ejaculations are good for them.

DEMYSTIFYING PROSTATITIS

When I have performed transrectal pelvic floor muscle assessments and prostate examinations on these patients, almost all of them have had tight and tender pelvic muscles. Their prostates also felt tight, congested (swollen) and tender. These men suffer from a type of prostatitis where they have a lot of inflammation in their prostate, which in turn, has led to the muscles around the prostate becoming inflamed and spastic (affected by muscle spasm). It does not matter at this point whether the infection is to blame but it is simply important to note that these men have worsening symptoms after ejaculation. If men with this type of prostatitis try to ejaculate more frequently, they provoke even more spasming, congestion and inflammation in their prostate and surrounding muscles.

All these mechanisms can be explained via knowledge of the physiology of the act of sex. Let me explain it in layman's terms.

A man experiences sexual arousal, leading to an erection and, eventually, climax with ejaculation. In simplified terms, this process is supported by increased blood flow to the penis, which leads to penile erection. At the same time, there is increased blood flow toward the prostate, seminal vesicles and muscles around the prostate (pubococcygeal muscles). The prostate becomes engorged with more fluid being secreted within. The surrounding muscles also become bulkier due to the increase of blood flow and an increase in their state of preparedness for contractions. During ejaculation all these entities contract to expel seminal fluid from the prostatic portion of the urethra. Moments later, the opposite effect takes place. There is a reduction in blood flow, and relaxation of the smooth muscles within the prostate and seminal vesicles, along with the relaxation of skeletal muscles within the pelvic floor complex. In basic terms, this is how the process goes for healthy men. Men who suffer from CP/CPPS often suffer a dysfunction of these mechanisms.

Regardless of whether men suffer bacterial or nonbacterial prostatitis, they experience an active inflammation within the prostate, and very often within the surrounding prostate fat tissue. It is also

DEMYSTIFYING PROSTATITIS

very common that pelvic muscles also become inflamed and therefore more contracted (spastic). If men suffer from CP for an extended period of time, the neural endings within the prostate and muscles surrounding the prostate also become inflamed (neurogenic inflammation).

When we perform Digital Rectal Examination (DRE) on these men, we often feel a congested, firm, and tender prostate. In addition, when we examine their pelvic floor muscles, they are often quite tender on palpation and feel spastic (contracted).

Now, let's see what happens when men with these types of problems try to ejaculate. We mentioned previously that during sexual arousal there is an increase in blood flow that takes place in the penis, prostate, seminal vesicles and surrounding muscles. They become more engorged with blood, the prostate secretes more fluid, and the surrounding muscles increase their tone. Once ejaculation takes place, the inflamed prostate does not contract and relax. Rather, it goes into a spasm and often stays this way for an extended period of time, which makes the prostate even more inflamed and congested.

This is why men feel more pain during and shortly after ejaculation. There is also a very similar process that takes place within the surrounding prostate muscles. They contract during ejaculation in order to facilitate ejection of seminal fluid, but they do not relax as quickly as they should under healthy conditions. For some men, they stay contracted, which also causes pain during and after ejaculations. Many men with CP/CPPS report weak force of ejaculation. They complain that their semen "leaks out" rather than shoots out on ejaculation. This phenomenon also occurs due to muscular dysfunction of smooth muscles within the prostate and the skeletal muscles of the pelvic floor complex.

There is another portion of muscular complex which often becomes hyperspastic in men with CP/CPPS. It is an external

DEMYSTIFYING PROSTATITIS

sphincter of the urethra, which is intimately close and attached to the capsule (a thin layer of connective tissue) of the prostate.

The external sphincter often goes into a state of excessive spasticity during and after ejaculation. Symptomatically it presents itself as feeling more urinary urgency and frequency after ejaculation. A hyperactive external sphincter can also cause a weaker force of ejaculation and a sensation of "blockage" during ejaculation. The latter is quite a common complaint by men with CP/CPPS. They fear having some kind of physical blockage near the prostate or within the urethra. Unless someone has significant scar tissue growth within the urethra, it is the external sphincter's over-spasticity that is responsible for the sensation of blockage on ejaculation.

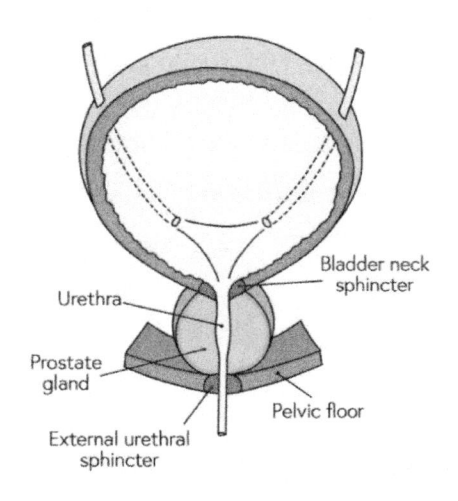

It is logical to conclude that men who suffer from the type of CP/CPPS described above will not benefit from frequent ejaculations. On the contrary, the more often they ejaculate the more symptoms they will experience. Hence, the recommendation to ejaculate frequently in their cases will be counterproductive and will make things worse for them, not better.

I have seen men who have discontinued every form of sex for months and even longer due to persistent pain. Nevertheless, many still continued practising regular masturbation despite enduring pain as a result. Needless to say, the whole process brought them no pleasure or satisfaction. On the contrary, it made matters worse not only on a physical level, but also contributed to increased anxiety and depression. Their sex drive declined, which in turn led to significant

DEMYSTIFYING PROSTATITIS

problems in their relationships with their existing partners and hindered the establishing of new relationships.

This is an extremely difficult problem for men to deal with. Unfortunately, health care providers are often not able to guide them effectively. I believe that education is the most effective approach to helping men with CP/CPPS who experience the above described problems. Men need to know why they experience pain and other symptoms around ejaculation. Once they are reassured that there is nothing too serious going on, they will feel less anxiety. Reassurance is a very significant factor in both reducing anxiety and muscular tension. It is not only inflammation in the prostate and surrounding muscles that triggers spasms and pain. Anxiety and stress make matters even worse. It is very common that men report an increase in their pain symptoms when they are more anxious and stressed. When it comes down to ejaculation, we cannot tell men to permanently abstain from ejaculation; it is simply unrealistic, especially for younger men.

If the symptoms are very intense, close to 8-10 on the VAS (Visual Analog Scale), then yes, it is better that men abstain from any kind of sexual activity until symptoms subside to an acceptable level. Once they are in a more manageable state, I will usually advise them to ejaculate with accepted frequency depending on their own needs. I do not endorse "must do" ejaculations under these circumstances. These are situations where men feel obliged to ejaculate because they feel it is supposed to be good for them, rather than being determined by their sex drive. If they are the type with a spastic prostate and spastic pelvic floor muscles, "mandatory" ejaculation will only worsen their condition. Also, if ejaculation is driven by necessity only, the erection will not be as strong as it would have been otherwise - which in turn only promotes more spasms, inflammation and, therefore, pain.

Another simple tactic which can help to reduce pain with ejaculation is heat. I often recommend that men with ejaculatory pain use heat in the form of a hot sitz bath or hot shower before they engage in sexual activity. It helps to relieve the pre-existing muscular tension in the pelvic area and decreases the intensity of pain afterwards. Of course, heat is advisable only if their symptoms stem from a chronic condition in the absence of significant infection.

Another piece of advice is to perform a lot of pelvic floor muscle stretching prior to and sometimes after ejaculation. This simple exercise will help to warm up the muscles and make them less spastic beforehand and reduce pain levels after ejaculation.

You have to understand that these are auxiliary recommendations. They are in no way a guarantee of resolution of pain or other symptoms related to ejaculation. They are only a part of the multimodal approach to treatment of CP/CPPS.

There is another group of men with CP/CPPS who report an improvement in their symptoms after ejaculation. They often present with the symptoms of feeling "heavy" in the prostate area, a sense of pressure and discomfort, and they tend to ejaculate much more frequently.

When I examine men with these characteristics, I often find that their prostate feels very soft, boggy, and that their pelvic floor muscle is rather sluggish. Prostate manipulation ("drainage") leads to a significant amount of prostatic fluid release. It is not uncommon for these men to report a substantial relief in their symptoms after prostate manipulation. These men typically suffer the type of CP where they have a reduced tonus of smooth muscles within the prostate along with reduced tone of the pelvic floor skeletal muscles. Frequent ejaculation in their case is not prohibited at all. Further, it is also possible to strengthen the skeletal muscles within the pelvic floor. The challenge remains how to make the prostate less boggy and how to improve the smooth muscles tonus within the prostate. Unfortunately, there is no drug which can reverse it, and there is no special exercise which can directly make the prostate less sluggish. The only effective solution to this problem is to have the prostate

DEMYSTIFYING PROSTATITIS

"drained" regularly in order to make it less bulky and reduce the amount of fluid it accumulates. I have seen men who managed to perform prostate self-manipulation ("massage") with various degrees of success. Health professionals with expertise in this field would be an asset to the process.

I have found this procedure especially beneficial when treating men with "boggy" prostates along with chronic bacterial infection in the prostate. A combination of antibiotics with very frequent prostate "drainages" have led to a significant resolution to many of their symptoms. Moreover, a significant number of our patients have been completely cured from this "dreadful" disease.

Dear readers, as you can see from this chapter, the ultimate question of "whether to ejaculate or not" remains an enigma. The answer to this question lies in the very nature of the CP/CPPS someone suffers. Each individual case must be looked at with care and consideration and managed accordingly. This is the case for the entirety of CP/CPPS condition. It requires hard work and commitment of both parties: the men themselves on one hand and the multidisciplinary health care team on another.

CHAPTER 7

Does size matter?

My dear readers! You are probably completely flabbergasted by the title of this chapter. What does size have to do with the story of prostatitis?

We are all very aware of this famous question, which has generated so many stories and jokes worldwide and has been a famous talking point for stand-up comedians. Men have always been preoccupied with the size of their penises. I do not think that I will be too far off to claim that the sexual organ is the most important organ to men. Many men would rather lose a limb than suffer from the malfunctioning or shrinking of their penis.

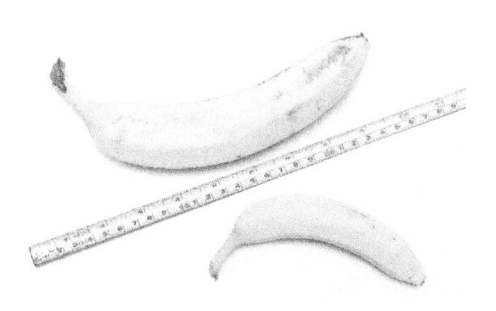

But we are not going to discuss penile matters in this chapter. The mere size of a penis has no relevance to the prostate and prostate related issues. The size of the *prostate*, however, does have relevance and is also on the mind of many men who suffer from prostate related symptoms. This is the size we will be discussing in this chapter.

Contrary to the penis, the prostate is an internal organ. Therefore, prostate size is not readily visible and is only relevant to the man to whom the prostate belongs. It is very well known in the medical community that as men grow older the prostate increases in size. The medical term for it is Benign Prostatic Hyperplasia or BPH. In lay terms we simply call it Prostate Enlargement.

DEMYSTIFYING PROSTATITIS

It has been reported that at many men over the age of 50 will have some degree of BPH[25]. And at least 90% of men after the age of 80 will suffer from this condition. It is very clear that BPH is an extremely common condition in men. So here we are, the most important point of the chapter. Does it matter whether you have an enlarged prostate or not? The answer is yes it does - but only if it causes you problems.

This is quite a twist for men's psyches. Men always want their penis larger, but the prostate smaller. There is probably not a single man in the whole world who would be upset about having a small prostate. On the contrary, when men learn they have a small prostate, they are elated and relieved. What is the reason for this? Well, men know that having an enlarged prostate almost always means potential problems with urination, among other complications.

As stated above, most men who develop BPH are over 45-50[26]. We also know that most men who suffer from chronic prostatitis are between ages 25 to 70.

So, as you can see, there is a significant population of men who may potentially suffer from both chronic prostatitis and BPH at the same time. This holds true in clinical practice. Most men over 50 that we have seen in our practice who suffer from CP also have had signs and symptoms of BPH. Both CP and BPH are interlaced in their effect on the prostate and the symptoms that cause men to suffer from these conditions.

Let's step back a little and look at younger men, aged 20 to 45, who suffer from CP. In previous chapters, we discussed in detail the signs and symptoms of CP.

One of the symptoms men often report is the feeling of swelling or enlargement in the prostate area triggered by either sexual activity, stress or various other factors. These are subjective symptoms men report to their doctor. They often believe that their prostate becomes enlarged when they experience these symptoms.

DEMYSTIFYING PROSTATITIS

When we perform diagnostic work, the most important test for men is the Digital Rectal Examination (DRE) of the prostate and surrounding muscles. When we examine men with DRE during their active flare up of CP, we often find that their prostate is swollen, congested, and tender on palpation. It does not mean that their prostate is actually enlarged as it is the case for BPH.

Younger men are often quite frantic about their prostate size. They often confuse the term "swelling" or "congestion" with the term "prostate enlargement". I will try to be as clear as possible here. When the prostate is inflamed it can become swollen, congested and, therefore, cause many symptoms such as pain, urinary frequency, urinary urgency, weaker urine flow, etc. When the inflammation subsides, the prostate becomes less congested, less swollen and, therefore, becomes completely normal in size. These are fluctuations in prostate size due to the severity of prostate inflammation.

By definition, we grade prostates being normal up to 25g in volume. The prostate is a 3-dimensional organ. That is why we measure its size either in grams or cubic centimeters (CC). Most men under the age of 45 have a normal size prostate. In the case of a man with active prostatitis, the prostate might feel swollen and congested, but is overall normal in size.

It is a different story for BPH. In the case of Benign Prostatic Hyperplasia, the prostate increases in size due to the growth of a benign tumour. It originates from a certain area of the prostate called the Transitional Zone located inside the prostate near the urethra.

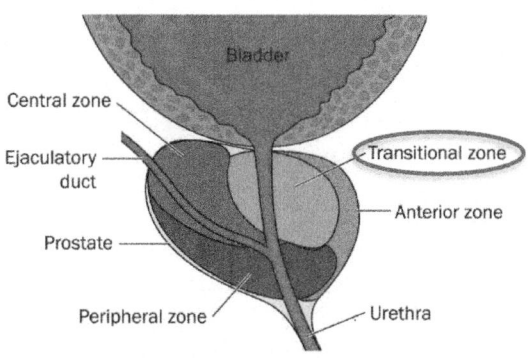

55

DEMYSTIFYING PROSTATITIS

It is not the whole prostate that increases in size. It is the growing benign tumour inside of the prostate that makes the overall prostate bigger. This benign tumor is encapsulated and also consists of tissues which are different from the rest of the actual prostate. This means that the actual BPH is separated from the rest of the prostate by a capsule. This is a very important point in understanding the relationship between BPH and chronic prostatitis.

Chronic prostatitis is an element of chronic inflammation and chronic infection affecting the actual prostate. In the case of men with BPH, the prostate is being "sandwiched" between the capsule of BPH from the inside and external capsule of the actual prostate itself. This anatomical feature defines clinical behaviour and symptoms in men who suffer both BPH and chronic prostatitis.

You can ask me a very fair question: How do we know what causes my symptoms? In order to answer this question, we need to look at the differences between typical symptoms of BPH and the symptoms of CP. Unfortunately, there are certain symptoms which overlap in both conditions.

Recall the most common symptoms of CP are:

- Pain or discomfort in the perineal, genital, pelvic area
- Urinary frequency, urgency, weaker urine flow, burning during or after urination, nocturia (need to urinate during sleep time)
- Sexual symptoms (erectile dysfunction, premature ejaculation, delayed ejaculation, pain during or after ejaculation, hematospermia (blood in semen)

What are the typical symptoms of BPH? Urinary symptoms only: urinary frequency, urinary urgency, weak urine flow, nocturia (nighttime urinary frequency), and inability to fully empty the bladder.

DEMYSTIFYING PROSTATITIS

These are the classic symptoms of BPH. As you can see, the symptoms of CP and BPH overlap only in one category and that is urinary symptoms.

It is important to note that men who suffer from BPH very often suffer from CP as well[27]. As a matter of fact, it is chronic prostatitis that often complicates the course of BPH behaviour. Do you remember the "sandwiched" prostate between two capsules? When the actual prostate is being "squeezed" due to BPH presence, it affects prostate physiology. It promotes inflammation and infection within the actual prostate. That is what often makes symptoms worse.

If you are a person with an enlarged prostate and you suffer from urinary symptoms but also experience symptoms of pain, discomfort, burning with or without urination, then you have a very strong chance of suffering CP at the same time. It is often prudent to treat the CP aspect of the problem in order to improve someone's condition overall.

The ability to identify CP and treat it in cases where men with BPH are heading for prostate surgery, especially TURP (Transurethral Resection of the Prostate), GreenLight Laser or PVP (Photoselective Vaporization of the Prostate), plays an important role in their post surgical recovery and the resolution of their symptoms.

Here is an example:

Mr. John Doe is a 67 year old man. He suffers from BPH and had a prostate that was 60g. He has had many urinary symptoms, including urinary frequency, urinary urgency, occasional burning on urination, and occasional pain and discomfort in the pelvic region. His urologist has treated him with a standard combination of Flomax and Avodart for a few years. Unfortunately, John continues to complain of the same symptoms which have had a substantial impact on his quality of life. The decision was made to perform a TURP. The surgery itself went without immediate complications. Within three months after the surgery, John started to experience more urinary

DEMYSTIFYING PROSTATITIS

symptoms, more pain than he had before. He also had a few episodes of urinary tract infection (UTI), and urinating lots of blood on a few occasions. He was treated with antibiotics by the same urologist without a permanent resolution of his symptoms.

Mr. Doe decided to seek help through our services. Upon examination, we discovered that his prostate was quite "boggy", "swollen", and very tender on manipulation. We released a significant amount of very infected prostatic fluid. Mr. Doe received an appropriate course of antibiotic treatment along with regular prostate "drainages" intended to decongest and debulk his prostate. This treatment has led to a complete resolution of his symptoms. He continues to do well one year after his initial visit.

We have seen quite a few men in a similar scenario to Mr. Doe after undergoing some type of prostate surgery. What is common in all these cases is that men have had BPH along with a chronic infection (chronic bacterial prostatitis) in their prostates. They all had surgery, either TURP or PVP, where very high temperatures were used to remove prostate tissue (BPH).

The "sandwich" effect described earlier enters into this scenario. This means that the actual prostate is literally being squeezed between two capsules and hosts colonies of semi-active bacteria. This chronically inflamed and infected prostate gets traumatized by high heat surgery. That is what often leads to an "explosion" of infection within the prostate and all of its consequences.

I am definitely not trying to talk you out of having surgical intervention of any type. If your BPH significantly impacts your quality of life or poses a significant health threat, you should follow your urologist's advice. I am simply making the important point that if you also have symptoms and signs of prostatitis at the same time, try to treat the prostatitis to the best of your doctor's ability to minimize possible complications after the surgery, should you choose to go that route. Nevertheless, please remember that surgery should be your last option. I believe that men should opt for surgery only after they have exhausted all other options and all other options failed. Once you have surgery on your prostate, you cannot undo it. There is a saying: "The best surgeon is the one who knows when not to operate".

Let's hope that there will be more men who would do well without surgery.

DEMYSTIFYING PROSTATITIS

CHAPTER 8

The biggest fear of all: Cancer

In the previous chapter we discussed matters related to the relationship between chronic prostatitis and BPH (prostate enlargement). There is yet another prostate condition to be discussed in terms of its relationship to CP, which is much more serious in terms of its health impact: prostate cancer.

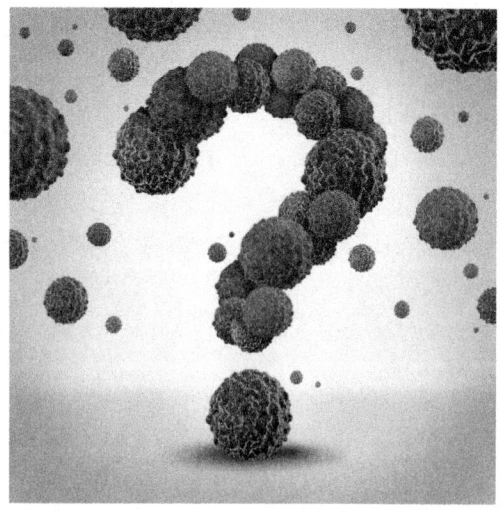

Prostate cancer is a serious disease. In its aggressive form, especially if not diagnosed early, it can be lethal. As a matter of fact, prostate cancer is the most common cancer in Canadian men (excluding non-melanoma skin cancers). According to the Canadian Cancer Society, it is the third leading cause of cancer-related death from cancer in Canadian men[28].

It is not my intention to devote this chapter specifically to prostate cancer. There is already a lot of easily accessible information about it on the internet on reputable websites. Also, there are a lot of books about it for both health care professionals and the public. Prostate cancer attracts a lot of attention in the media due to its significance as a public health issue.

Prostate cancer is a major concern and is on the mind of many men who suffer from chronic prostatitis. Unfortunately, we do not often hear nor read about how chronic prostatitis relates to prostate cancer, or if and when there is a connection between these two conditions.

DEMYSTIFYING PROSTATITIS

Many men with symptoms of CP suffer great anxiety directly caused by the fear of cancer. It is not enough that their quality of life is already dismal due to the relentless daily symptoms they endure; their situation is significantly worsened by this growing fear of something much worse. It is unfortunate that this anxiety caused by the assumption that symptoms of CP means cancer is never discussed or even referred to in the media, literature or on major health-related websites.

Let me remind you that chronic prostatitis is the most common urological condition in men aged 18 to 65. Hundreds of thousands of men worldwide live with this condition. And many of these men, due to fear and misinformation, believe they have cancer and suffer in great fear and anxiety. Even worse, many of them are often forced to suffer in silence. These men are either reluctant to discuss it with their health providers, or they do not even have one. They often turn to the internet for answers, but do not know how to interpret what they have read.

I have seen many men in our clinic who expressed concerns about prostate cancer. Many of them were not only concerned about developing prostate cancer in the future, but they were actually concerned that they already *had* prostate cancer because many of their symptoms matched the symptoms of prostate cancer. The majority of these patients were young men who did not have prostate cancer but truly believed their symptoms aligned with those listed online.

We have had long discussions with these men to educate them about prostate cancer and prostatitis, providing reassurance and enforcing positive thinking. Many men require reassurance on multiple visits, simply because they still have had a hard time overcoming this anxiety.

Why do so many men with CP fear prostate cancer? I personally believe it is due to a lack of knowledge and understanding of both conditions.

DEMYSTIFYING PROSTATITIS

As you have previously read, CP usually affects younger men aged 18 to 65. Nonetheless, it is definitely possible for men over the age of 65 to have prostatitis. But men over the age of 65 are definitely more likely to suffer from BPH (prostate enlargement) and prostate cancer. It is important to point out that there are rare cases where men in their forties or even younger have developed prostate cancer, but these are statistically small numbers. We will try to focus here on the majority of men, so we do not get lost in individual cases. As you can see here, there is an age overlap from 50 to 65 where men can possibly have both conditions, chronic prostatitis and prostate cancer.

Does prostatitis cause prostate cancer? This is a legitimate concern among prostatitis sufferers. Honestly, it is a million-dollar question to which, to date, nobody has found a definite answer. This is largely due no doubt to the fact that there has not been a lot of research dedicated to this particular subject.

Anatomically, we know that the Peripheral Zone of the prostate is most likely to be affected by both prostatitis and prostate cancer.

There are research publications studying different pro-inflammatory markers which have been found in both prostate tissues affected by inflammation and prostate cancer. Nevertheless, when we review clinical studies looking into the correlation between CP (Chronic Prostatitis), BPH (Benign Prostatic Hyperplasia) and prostate cancer, most of these studies come to the conclusion that CP is more likely to cause BPH than prostate cancer in older men[29, 30].

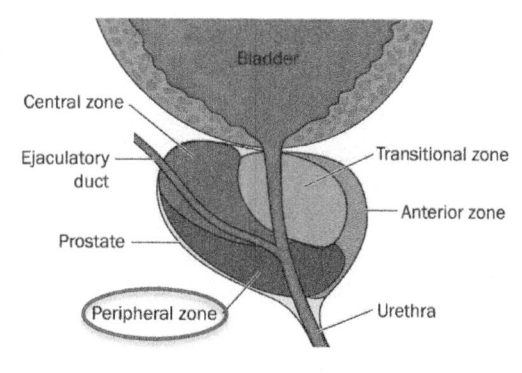

DEMYSTIFYING PROSTATITIS

Many prominent urologists who specialize in prostate cancer research and treatment are also split in their opinions. We definitely know one thing: more research is needed.

We know that prostatitis is a very common condition in younger men. We also know that the majority of men over the age of 65 develop BPH. It is also estimated that 1 in 9 men will develop prostate cancer and 1 in 29 men will die from it[31]. There are many other factors which lead to BPH and prostate cancer development. Unfortunately, to this day we are still in the research phase of establishing with certainty what these factors are.

A lot of research has been conducted in the field of genetic mutations at the chromosomal level as potential causes of prostate cancer. Again, the prostatitis connection is still uncertain.

It is important to emphasize that prostate cancer, unless it is an extremely aggressive form, develops slowly. When prostate cancer is in its early stages of development, and therefore completely confined within the prostate gland, it does not cause any symptoms. This is in juxtaposition to prostatitis, which is a condition literally based on symptoms. The only reason we diagnose men with prostatitis is because they present themselves with various symptoms. In most industrialized countries, men generally see their primary care physician at least once per year. If you are 50 years old or older, there is a good chance that you've had a DRE (Digital Rectal Examination) of your prostate and/or PSA (Prostate Specific Antigen) blood test as part of the screening for prostate cancer. If both these parameters were always normal and you suddenly developed symptoms indicative of prostatitis, there is an extremely high chance that it is prostatitis.

I would like to emphasize another "twist of fortune". Men who suffer from chronic prostatitis are much less likely to be diagnosed with late stage prostate cancer due to the simple fact that they see either their General Practitioner or Urologist much more frequently.

DEMYSTIFYING PROSTATITIS

Therefore, they get their prostates examined and PSA tests done regularly.

If you have been to a doctor regarding your prostatitis symptoms, and if you have had your prostate examined and have had your PSA test done without any worrisome comments from your doctor, you have nothing to worry about.

On the contrary, men in their 50's or older who have never had a prostate examination and never had a PSA test, should make an effort to do both. Prostate cancer, like many other cancers, is completely silent until it spreads outside of its boundaries. Therefore, its early detection is only possible through proactive screening procedures.

Here, I would like to focus more specifically on the PSA test.

The PSA abbreviation means Prostate Specific Antigen. It is a form of protein which is produced in abundance by the prostate gland. Therefore, prostatic fluid and seminal fluid contain very high levels of this protein. Only a very small fraction of this protein gets into the blood.

The levels of PSA in blood may increase not only due to cancer, but also due to BPH (Benign Prostatic Hyperplasia) and prostatitis.

There has been a lot of controversy lately around PSA testing and its interpretation. Yes, I agree that interpreting elevated levels of PSA might be very challenging. It is something that should be left to Urologists. PSA interpretation should be done in correlation with many other factors: age, DRE of the prostate, symptomatology and previous PSA values. Basically, PSA is not just a number to be taken at face value.

I have noticed lately that there is a trend among Primary Care physicians to use PSA as a test for prostatitis. I have seen many men with signs and symptoms of prostatitis in their early 30's who have had a PSA test done by their General Practitioners intentionally as a tool to diagnose prostatitis. There is absolutely no merit in doing this test in young men. PSA is a test only for prostate cancer screening.

DEMYSTIFYING PROSTATITIS

By the way, the majority of these men have had completely normal PSA values despite having chronic prostatitis symptoms. But there is another risk in doing PSA tests in men with prostatitis. When men have an acute phase of prostate infection, their PSA levels are usually much higher than their baseline. It is a very common phenomenon. That is why we usually avoid doing tests for PSA during an acute phase of prostatitis. Elevated levels of PSA recorded at that time often trigger unnecessary anxiety in these men and require retesting, sometimes more then once. As a result, what we have here are men who are already stressed due to their prostate problems becoming even more stressed due to abnormal PSA levels, and unnecessary health care expenses.

My dear readers, if you have all the signs of an active infection in your prostate, and you happen to have an elevated PSA registered during that time, please calm down. Just wait a few weeks or more until your prostate condition settles down and only then ask your doctor to recheck your PSA.

There is another group of men which deserve special attention: those with Asymptomatic Prostatitis.

These men are mostly 50 years of age or older. They visit their doctors for regular check ups, they usually have a prostate that is larger than normal, but their PSA values are much higher than they should be for their age and prostate size. It is important to emphasize that these men typically have no symptoms of active prostatitis, maybe just mild urinary symptoms caused by prostate enlargement. These men usually end up having a prostate biopsy completed to rule out cancer and the biopsy pathology report comes back negative for cancer. These men continue to monitor their PSA every few months. PSA levels remain high, or even climb higher. They are subjected to another biopsy, which is negative as well. Many of these men, if they live in big cities, have Prostate MRIs done (Prostate Magnetic Resonance Imaging), which find no cancer.

DEMYSTIFYING PROSTATITIS

Let me present you with this example:

Mr. John Doe, a 54 year old Caucasian man was referred to a Prostatitis Clinic for assessment. He presented with no symptoms of prostatitis. John reported having elevated levels of PSA between 8 to 10 ng/ml (normal levels are between 0 to 3.5 ng/mL) over the last 5 years, which led to having four prostate biopsies. None of the biopsies showed prostate cancer, but prostate inflammation was reported in a few samples.

On DRE his prostate was very soft, enlarged, "boggy" and moderately tender. Upon prostate manipulation, we managed to release a significant amount of prostatic fluid. Direct microscopy of this fluid yielded numerous white blood cells and other entities typical for chronic prostate infection. John was treated with a prolonged course of antibiotics along with regular prostate manipulations. After completion of this treatment, his PSA level substantially decreased to an acceptable baseline, and his prostate cancer worries were put to rest.

As you can see, John is one of many men who have elevated PSA due to "silent" prostatitis. This is an example of how complex an interpretation of PSA might be.

I am not trying to persuade you to be totally ignorant of the possibility of having prostate cancer. On the contrary, every man who is older than 45 should be screened for it by means of a PSA test and digital rectal examination.

I would warn you, though, that there are some physicians who prefer to perform PSA tests only and abolish physical examination of the prostate altogether. I personally believe this to be a big mistake. Not every prostate cancer leads to elevated PSA. There are very aggressive prostate cancers which do not cause a rise in PSA. That is the reason why every man, after a certain age, should have a prostate examination done as well. Men who have a very strong family history of prostate cancer (father, siblings), or breast cancer on their maternal

DEMYSTIFYING PROSTATITIS

side (mother, siblings), should commence prostate cancer screening at age 35.

I hope that I have not made you more confused than you were before. I have tried to show you how complex the relationship between prostatitis and prostate cancer can be. Many men have both prostatitis and prostate cancer simultaneously and through meticulous assessment and treatment, we are able to diagnose them with being in the early stages of prostate cancer.

I do want to remind you that if you have prostatitis symptoms, it is most likely due to prostatitis. Please stay calm and focused on the diagnosis and treatment of this disease. If you are at the age where you need to be screened for prostate cancer, do it with the utmost diligence, and have your doctor engaged in this process to the best of his professional abilities.

I hope you are not too tired and stressed after reading this chapter. Please take a break, go for a walk, or do something cheerful.

We will meet again soon... at the next chapter!

CHAPTER 9

How do you like your Head - With the Helmet or Without?

You're probably reading the title of this chapter and likely chuckling because you know exactly what I'm referring to.

Yes, you guessed it. I am talking about the penis - circumcised or uncircumcised.

You are likely asking a very legitimate question: "What does the presence or absence of a foreskin on the penis have to do with prostatitis?" My answer is: "quite often a lot".

Let me clarify. Obviously, whether a man is circumcised or not has no specific bearing on prostatitis as a medical condition. There are thousands of men, both circumcised and uncircumcised, who suffer equally from the negative effect of prostatitis. The types of prostatitis which men develop, and their clinical presentations and treatments, are pretty much the same in both categories.

The reason I decided to dedicate a separate chapter, albeit small, to the subject of extra skin on the penis is because it often makes a difference whether prostatitis develops in men in the first place.

The mere presence of skin covering the head of the penis is not a concern. Having an uncircumcised penis does not increase the risk of developing prostatitis. What does increase the risk of prostatitis is when uncircumcised men develop problems with their foreskin (the skin flap that covers the Glans Penis/penile head).

Let me present to you one of these cases:

An 18 year old man came to our clinic with a classic presentation of chronic prostatitis. He was complaining of low-level pain in the genital area and perineum, burning, irritation along urethra, and some

DEMYSTIFYING PROSTATITIS

low-level pain during and after ejaculation. He had experienced these symptoms for more than a year. It is worthwhile noting that in discussing the history of his symptoms, it yielded no "red flags". There was nothing in the young man's past life that would explain why he developed prostatitis in the first place. It is important to note that this young man had never had sexual contact with another person. He practiced only masturbation on a regular basis. His masturbation technique, as it was described to us, was within normal practice. Basically, his overall health, sexual habits and lifestyle gave us no clues as to why he developed prostatitis.

Now, we approach an important moment: the physical examination. Let me jump forward a little bit. Prostate examination and Expressed Prostatitis Secretion (EPS) analysis confirmed chronic prostatitis with signs of infection within the prostate gland. A focused examination of the penis revealed that the young man had phimosis (very tight foreskin). The glans of the penis could not be exposed. Also, there were signs of chronic infection and inflammation around the urethral opening (meatus), skin of the glans penis and foreskin (balanoposthitis).

Bingo!!! Now we know what the cause of prostatitis was in this young man's case.

It is important to understand that men develop prostatitis due to one cause or another. The most common cause of prostatitis is infection, especially in younger men. The infection has to get into the prostate from somewhere. In this particular case, the only source of infection was phimosis. The sebaceous glands around the glans developed smegma (a thick, white, cheesy substance). In the case of phimosis, smegma accumulates between the foreskin and the head of the penis and cannot be effectively washed off. This type of environment creates an ideal condition for all kinds of organisms, both bacterial and fungal, to thrive. Due to the immediate proximity to the urethral meatus, organisms can easily enter the urethra and gradually find their way up into the prostate.

DEMYSTIFYING PROSTATITIS

This is exactly what happened with our young man. The good news is that after undergoing the appropriate treatment with antibiotics and the implementation of thorough hygienic practices around the head of the penis, he was cured from prostatitis and balanoposthitis.

What was astonishing about this particular case was that this young man was completely oblivious to what was happening around his penis. He practiced masturbation regularly. The head of his penis had never been exposed during erection. He observed smegma discharge on a regular basis, and also saw redness on the foreskin and around the meatus. Nevertheless, he never thought that there was anything wrong with this appearance. Only after he developed symptoms of prostatitis did he decide to seek professional help. What was even more astonishing that this young man was seen by at least one or two doctors, neither of whom brought the phimosis to his attention, or identified it as being a potential problem.

This is not an unusual case. We have seen quite a few men with various degrees of phimosis complicated by local infection who eventually developed prostatitis.

The main point of this chapter is to emphasize the importance of maintaining good hygienic practices around the genital area, the penis, and the foreskin in particular. This recommendation applies to all men. For circumcised men to practice good penile hygiene is relatively easy. It is recommended that the penile area be washed regularly, ideally with running water and a small amount of soap.

Men who are not circumcised should take a much more vigorous approach to the hygienic care of their foreskin and head of the penis. Uncircumcised men have a much higher risk of developing balanoposthitis (inflammation of the foreskin and penile head), which can potentially cause prostatitis due to the infectious contamination of the urethra. Therefore, when uncircumcised men wash their penile area, they should always retract the foreskin all the way back during washing, otherwise it is useless.

Men with phimosis should pay utmost attention to their penile hygiene since they present the highest risk of carrying a chronic infection around the head of the penis, which can become the cause of prostate infection. Since they cannot retract the foreskin all the way, it is practically impossible to achieve a full hygienic wash around the head of the penis. Some men with phimosis even utilize a small syringe to flush water under the foreskin in the attempt to wash smegma off. A small note concerning the best soap to use for these types of washes: I strongly recommend avoiding using any liquid soaps. First of all, they often contain additional chemicals such as preservatives and at the same time lack antiseptic abilities. Also, try to avoid perfumed soaps for the same reason. The more plain the soap, the better it is for the penile area and the less chance it has of causing chemical irritation on the skin. Overall, use soap sparingly and primarily use running lukewarm water. If the skin in that area is prone to being too dry, use a small amount of oil-based product, or perhaps even a small amount of Vaseline.

Here we approach an enigmatic question: to circumcise or not to circumcise.

The issue of circumcision has been a controversial subject for many years. There are different reasons why men are circumcised. They can be divided into three categories: religious, cultural, and medical.

I am not going to discuss religious and cultural circumcisions. They have no relevance to the subject we are discussing here. No matter what controversies surround the subject of cultural circumcision, one thing is very clear to me: circumcised men will never develop phimosis and they have a much lower risk of developing infection and inflammation around the penile head. It is also scientifically proven that circumcised men have a much lower risk of developing penile cancer and contracting HIV in heterosexual men.

I am not trying to promote circumcision. This is a choice that parents make for their baby boys or that men make for themselves. There are cultural and religious groups which will prohibit circumcision no matter what. It is, obviously, their choice to make.

There is also medical circumcision. It is performed in cases of phimosis.

I have seen grown men with phimosis complicated by balanoposthitis and prostatitis. Unfortunately, they have a lot of issues on their hands. Nonetheless, we treated and resolved their prostatitis. We often managed to keep balanoposthitis under good control as well. Phimosis typically cannot be resolved without surgery. There are men who have partial phimosis. They can retract their foreskin, but not all the way beyond the penile head. These men are often able to completely reverse their phimosis by regularly practising foreskin stretching and maintaining vigorous hygienic practices.

On the other hand, if phimosis is complete and foreskin retraction is not possible, circumcision remains the only option.

There are adult men with severe phimosis who are really fearful of circumcision. Please, let's be realistic here. Think about your options: either you live for the rest of your life with severe phimosis, which often leads to complications such as balanoposthitis, prostatitis, an increased risk of penile cancer and HIV, or, you have a simple circumcision which will absolve you of many possible problems mentioned here. Obviously, circumcision is a surgical procedure that carries a small risk of some local complications. If you have it done by a licensed urologist, the benefits of circumcision much outweigh its risks.

My dear readers, at this point I would like to make an appeal to all parents with young boys.

DEMYSTIFYING PROSTATITIS

If you are not part of a religious or cultural group which would have your baby boy circumcised shortly after his birth, please pay close attention to your son's foreskin. Every so often, when you bathe your son, try to make sure that their foreskin is healthy looking and not tight. Please make sure that the penile area is being carefully washed on a regular basis. If at some point, you consistently notice that the foreskin is tight, does not retract, take your son to see his doctor. If a diagnosis of phimosis is confirmed, having a circumcision done at a much younger age is so much easier to recover from. Having a young boy with phimosis circumcised at a younger age will save him from much potential grief in his adulthood.

Please think about what was discussed in this chapter and make a wise decision.

Now, my dear readers, let's take another break and then move on to the next chapter.

CHAPTER 10

Sorry if you love beer

This chapter will be the most disliked chapter in this book. We are not going to discuss the symptoms or the management of prostatitis. Instead, we are going to discuss the lifestyle of men who suffer from prostatitis.

It is a well-established truth that lifestyle habits have a significant impact on many health-related issues such as diabetes, high blood pressure, hypercholesterolemia (elevated cholesterol), mood disorders, and many others.

Chronic prostatitis is no exception to this list. On the contrary, symptoms of CP are often affected by men's lifestyles: what men eat, drink or do on a daily basis often affects how they feel. After all, CP is a chronic inflammatory condition. Therefore, inflammation is often affected by lifestyle habits. The overwhelming majority of men who suffer from CP report a worsening of their symptoms after either drinking or eating something, or after certain physical activities, or after inactivity.

We are going to dig deeper into these lifestyle habits, so you, get a better understanding of the relationship between CP and lifestyle habits.

It is important to emphasize that lifestyle does not always affect symptoms of prostatitis. This is particularly true of men who suffer from an active form of infection in the prostate. During this phase, men often continue to experience the same symptoms despite being on their best behaviour. Nevertheless, lifestyle does have a significant impact on the progression of chronic prostatitis and the ability of CP sufferers to achieve long term remission, or even a potential cure.

We can divide lifestyle behaviours into four categories:

DEMYSTIFYING PROSTATITIS

- Food consumption
- Liquid consumption
- Physical activity (or lack thereof)
- Sexual behaviour

When it comes to food and liquid consumption, I generally try to divide them into two categories: pro-inflammatory and anti-inflammatory.

As an aside, I am not reinventing the wheel here. There are many publications on anti-inflammatory diets, many of which are quite extreme and difficult to sustain. Also, I do not believe that extreme diets are generally beneficial, at least in cases of chronic prostatitis. I personally believe in a more sensible approach to dietary lifestyles, which are generally more sustainable and therefore yield more benefits in the long term.

It is important to note, as well, that there is a significant variation in men's reactions to certain food products. So, with that in mind, the purpose of this chapter is to provide men with guidelines, rather than strict directives.

It is easier and less time consuming to list food products that are not recommended than those that are. Nowadays, we often live in multicultural communities and as a result, many men are exposed to a great variety of cuisines. What do we know from empirical experience and scientific data regarding what food men should avoid?

Foods

Spicy food

Men who report a worsening of their symptoms often do so after consuming spicy food. They also commonly report a worsening of their symptoms after eating out rather than eating at home.

When you order a meal at a restaurant, you have much less control over what has been added to your order. Please note, that when we say spicy food, we mean SPICY food and not spices. Spicy food may contain peppers such as jalapeno, serrano, hot chili peppers and black peppers. If you order a meal that comes with salsa, hot sauce or black pepper, you may have to ride out another flare up of CP symptoms. If you are a regular consumer of Indo-Asian cuisine, your taste buds are used to spicy food. This means to feel that kick, you're more likely to consume even "hotter" foods without realising it.

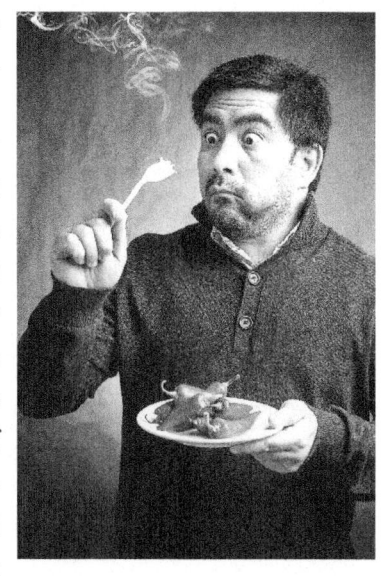

Regular spices such as ginger, garlic, cinnamon, cumin, cloves, onions, nutmeg and many others are generally not a problem. Many spices actually possess anti-inflammatory effects and their regular use is rather to be encouraged. On the other hand, with the possible exception of hotter spices like paprika, wasabi and hot curries are not generally a problem. I am not suggesting that you should avoid hotter spices or even spicy food altogether, but I usually recommend following a simple rule: use them sparingly and watch your symptoms. If you begin to consume something and suddenly you begin to feel a flare up of symptoms, stop consuming it and avoid it as much as possible. If you feel fine, you can continue to eat it, judiciously, in small quantities and infrequently.

Dairy products

Milk based products and whether they should be avoided due to their possible pro-inflammatory effect remains controversial. It has been suggested that the protein casein, which is found in milk, can be responsible for inducing inflammation. Personally, I do not have a

DEMYSTIFYING PROSTATITIS

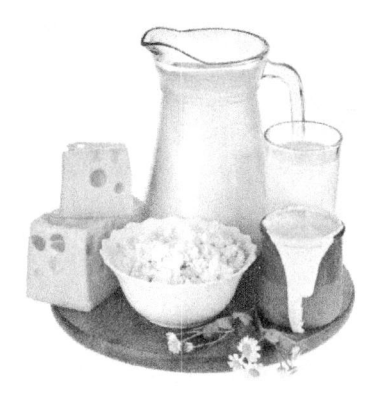

definitive answer to the issue of whether milk products are to be avoided or not.

There are men who are lactose intolerant or who develop allergies to casein. These men will, naturally, abstain from using dairy products. I usually recommend avoiding drinking milk, especially if it is consumed in large quantities such as a glass or more per day. I find that milk products such as plain yogurt, cottage cheese, mild cheese, or kefir do not generally have any negative impact on symptoms of chronic prostatitis.

It is important to mention that there are many men who suffer both chronic prostatitis (CP) and Irritable Bowel Syndrome (IBS) simultaneously. These men often experience symptoms of IBS after consuming certain dairy products or spicy foods. Many symptoms of IBS also overlap with symptoms of CP (low abdominal pains, urinary symptoms). For these men, avoidance of dairy products is logical for both reasons.

As far as CP is concerned, dairy fat has no impact on prostate inflammation. On the other hand, low fat dairy usually contains more processed milk products and more sugar to compensate for the loss of taste. Processed milk products and sugar possess a pro-inflammatory effect and so when it comes to dairy products, my general recommendation is to avoid low fat dairy.

Also, avoid dairy with added flavors, because it means sugar has been added. You also need to be aware that we need to consume good fat. Fat is an important source of energy storage for long-term use. In addition, fat is a type of chemical which is necessary for the synthesis of hormones, and for processing many different vitamins; it is an essential component of brain tissue and bone marrow, and is essential in many other important body functions. Therefore, the take home message is that if you like to consume dairy, stick to high fat. That being said, overall dairy consumption should be kept to a minimum as far as an anti-inflammatory diet is concerned.

Sugar

Sugar is one of the most significant pro-inflammatory food products which will affect prostatitis sufferers. The most significant product is refined sugar. It is not only empirical knowledge but also scientifically proven that refined sugars promote inflammation in the human body. It is not a prostate specific feature. Refined sugar promotes inflammation in many organs, tissues and arterial blood vessels, and since we are discussing chronic prostatitis, it is highly relevant to this condition. Men often report a flare of their symptoms after consumption of food and liquids high in sugar.

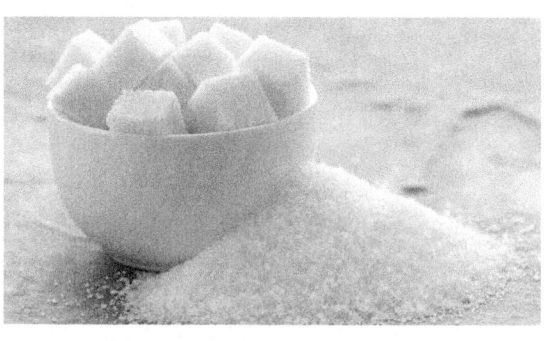

It is fair to state that it is practically impossible to completely avoid refined sugar. Refined sugar is present in most food products which are subjected to processing.

Again, I usually recommend using common sense in your food choices. When it comes to refined sugar, I usually advise avoiding eating candies, pastries, ice cream, cakes and sugary drinks, like commercial fruit juices and soft drinks, and, of course, avoiding sugar itself.

You are probably thinking: What is there left to indulge in?

Some examples of sweet foods you can still enjoy in small quantities are dark chocolate (cacao content of 60% or higher), fresh fruit of any type, small amounts of pure honey, or pure maple syrup. If you eat something with refined sugar once in a blue moon, in small

DEMYSTIFYING PROSTATITIS

quantities, it is acceptable. It is how much and how often you consume prohibited foods that makes a difference.

Processed foods

Any food item which has been subjected to a mechanical or chemical operation belongs to a group of processed foods. Practically speaking, that means that any food that is packaged in a jar, bag or box and contains some preservatives count as processed foods. Any cured meat in the form of cold cuts, sausage, bacon, or pastrami, for example, are processed and either contain additional chemicals, or have been subjected to thermal treatment.

It has been postulated and scientifically proven that processed foods contain pro-inflammatory properties. This includes red meat, especially if it has been cooked on a grill. We discourage our patients from eating processed foods due to their pro-inflammatory effect. Needless to say, the pro-inflammatory effect of processed foods is harmful to the whole body and is also harmful to the prostate, especially when the prostate is already inflamed in the case of chronic prostatitis.

The fewer trips you make to fast food restaurants, the better. The less white bread you consume, the better. The less fried food you consume, the better. Try to stay away from foods high in carbs, such as white potatoes, white rice, and white pasta.

Please do not get upset that I am taking all of your favourite foods away. I am not suggesting completely eliminating this food from your diet, but to keep in mind that moderation is the key to everything. If you go to your favourite fast food restaurant once every few weeks or months, you are still doing well. If you do it a few times per week, we may have a problem. Think about your long-term overall health and prostate health. Do the right thing and you will not regret it.

The take home message would be that the more natural and least processed food (made from scratch, if you will) that you consume, the better off you will be. When you buy food in a box or jar or other package, read the ingredients, not just the calories. If the label lists ingredients that do not exist in nature, it's best to avoid it. Use your common sense and consume everything in moderation. The human body does not like extremes. Keep everything in balance; this is the long-term solution for an anti-inflammatory diet.

Now, let's talk about liquids - what is advisable to drink and what is not.

Liquids

Water

Water is obviously a BIG yes. We all have to drink water. The question that often arises is how much water we should be drinking. Unfortunately, there is no universal answer to this question. It is often quoted by health authorities that we should all aim for eight 8 oz glasses of water per day. However, to some individuals, consuming this amount of water per day can and does exacerbate their condition, especially given that we get our "recommended" daily intake of water from other foods and beverages we consume regularly throughout the day. In this case, adding an additional eight 8oz glasses of water would be a significant amount.

I have seen many men with CP who reported significant urinary symptoms such as urinary frequency and urgency. They often significantly limit their water consumption in an attempt to curb their symptoms. They often complain that if they drink more than a litre of water per day, they are constantly running to the washroom to urinate. And so, we are faced with a conundrum here.

On one hand, men with CP need to drink more water in order to help reduce prostate inflammation. On the other hand, drinking more water worsens their urinary symptoms.

The treatment of CP, and its complications, are supposed to improve urinary symptoms. Limitation of water intake is not a problem solver. I usually encourage my patients to gradually increase their water intake up to an average of 1.5 to 2 litres per day.

DEMYSTIFYING PROSTATITIS

It is always better to drink water frequently, but in small volumes in order to facilitate its better absorption and metabolism. I often also recommend drinking previously boiled lukewarm water with a small amount of lemon and apple cider vinegar, if your stomach tolerates it. These additions to regular water promote anti-inflammatory effects in the body.

Now, what about other liquids?

Coffee

Many men with chronic prostatitis report a worsening of their symptoms if they drink too much coffee. It has been assumed that the caffeine in coffee has a detrimental and pro-inflammatory effect on CP.

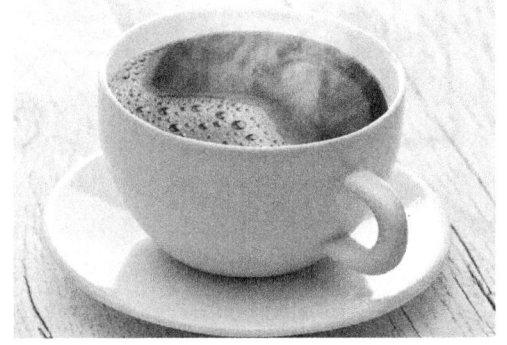

On the other hand, coffee has its health benefits as well. If you're someone who loves drinking coffee, one coffee per day after breakfast should be fine. Also, avoid milk in coffee. Drink it after breakfast, not on an empty stomach, as drinking it on an empty stomach will result in a much more rapid absorption. You will have a rush of caffeine into your bloodstream and, therefore, a much stronger negative impact on the prostate. Alternatively, some men switch to decaffeinated coffee and tolerate it well.

Men who are not fans of coffee or cannot tolerate coffee at all may turn to other beverages, such as tea. There is not as much of a problem with drinking tea, as long as these teas contain small amounts of caffeine and tannins. It's important to be aware that many teas, especially black tea and green tea, can contain as much caffeine as coffee. Tannins in tea are also a subject of controversy in terms of its health effects on the human body. I would recommend taking the same approach to tea as you would to coffee. One to two cups of tea per day, without sugar or milk, should be acceptable. Please

DEMYSTIFYING PROSTATITIS

remember that the only real refined sugar substitute is naturally derived sugar, such as in honey or maple syrup. I advise men to be cautious about using artificial sweeteners because they contain chemicals with pro-inflammatory properties.

Again, please remember the foundation of this chapter: moderation and sticking to basics.

Fruit juices

I recommend keeping your juice intake to a minimum due to high sugar content. What I'm referring to more specifically are regular processed juices (not necessarily freshly squeezed juices). Regular commercial juices have a much higher sugar content and are therefore more likely to promote inflammation. If you are a really big fan of juice, I would suggest keeping your intake to a maximum of 1-2 small glasses per day. Of course, water still reigns as king.

Alcohol

Most men consume alcohol in small and moderate amounts. There is also a great variation in types of alcohol being consumed. We have many choices: spirits (vodka, whiskey, gin, brandy, rum, tequila), wine (red, white), liquors and the most infamous, beer.

There is an overall consensus among medical professionals that alcoholic beverages are not recommended for men with chronic prostatitis because they promote inflammation. There is, however, a variation in men's reaction to alcohol.

I absolutely agree with the consensus that the less alcohol men drink, the less inflammation it promotes in the prostate. Many men with CP are still very keen on drinking alcohol for various reasons and want to know which type of alcohol is safest for them to drink. I may not be able to tell you which alcohol is best to drink, but I can tell you with one hundred percent certainty that in terms of alcohol consumption beer has the worst effect of inflammation in the prostate.

DEMYSTIFYING PROSTATITIS

Beer is a very common drink among men in Canada. When I review the lifestyles of my new patients and advise them of the trouble with beer intake, they are enormously surprised.

Most men with CP identify a flare up of symptoms specifically after drinking beer. It is still unknown why in particular beer is so bad for men with CP. As you would logically think, beer has a much smaller alcohol content (a maximum of 6%) in comparison to spirits. So, it is not the alcohol itself that triggers most of the inflammation in the prostate. There are speculations that it may be due to the live yeast and/or hops in the beer that are responsible for promoting inflammation in the prostate.

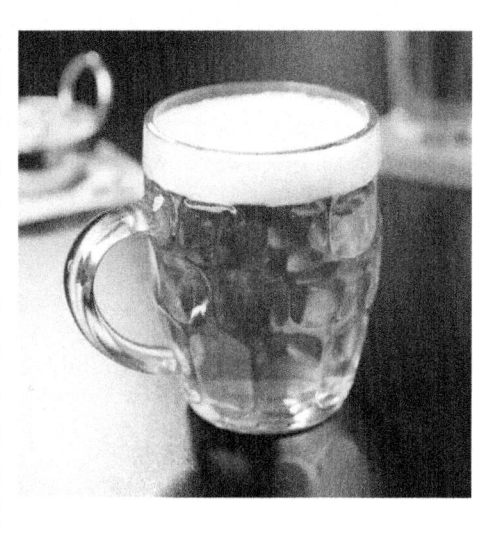

I have seen many men with CP who drink vodka or whiskey without any flare up of symptoms. Some men even feel better after drinking spirits. It does not necessarily mean that you should drink more than you already do, as these are anecdotal reports. Universally, it is definitely best to stay away from beer. Again, if you have a maximum of one beer every few months, it is not a big problem. If you have a habit of drinking beer weekly, you should seriously reconsider and drastically slow down.

Here is one example:

Mike, a 56 year old professional, came to the clinic with a long history of chronic prostatitis. He presented mostly with bothersome symptoms of urinary frequency and urgency. He had been treated with antibiotics in the past without significant effect. The main highlight of his lifestyle habits was beer drinking. He had been

DEMYSTIFYING PROSTATITIS

drinking 1 - 2 regular beers per day. His prostate assessment revealed no signs of infection.

I encouraged him to drastically cut down on his beer intake but was faced with very strong skepticism in regard to this recommendation. Mike, instead, opted for taking some herbal supplements. One month later, when we met again, Mike continued to report the same symptoms. I challenged him about beer drinking again and he finally committed to a one-month cessation of beer drinking (to start) and then we would reassess whether any change in symptoms had taken place. Lo and behold, one month later, Mike hadn't changed anything about his lifestyle except cessation of beer consumption but admitted that his symptoms were ninety percent better. He was astonished and happy to be feeling better.

Mike's case is an extreme one, but I have personally received positive feedback from many other patients who observed a reduction in their symptoms after no longer drinking beer.

Other alcoholic beverages can also have a negative impact on men with chronic prostatitis. It seems the sugar content has a role in this as well. The higher the sugar content in alcohol, the more likely it will upset the prostate. Therefore, liqueurs, fortified wines, rums and other beverages will have a negative impact on CP. If mixed drinks are more to your taste, you are more likely to drink something with much higher sugar content and therefore experience a flare up.

There are a lot of variations in men's responses to different alcoholic beverages, so these are general recommendations which I believe most men with chronic prostatitis should follow. Please remember that drinking alcohol and eating problematic foods together will double your risk of flare up of inflammation in the prostate.

I want, once more, to remind you that these lifestyle changes, such as eating healthy and drinking sensibly, will have a positive impact in the long term, not only for your prostate, but for your health overall. If you have an active infection in your prostate, a healthy dietary

DEMYSTIFYING PROSTATITIS

lifestyle might not provide you with immediate relief until your infection is under control, but I still strongly advise you to follow it. You need to create an anti-inflammatory environment for your prostate so it can heal from inflammation in the long run.

Let us move on to another important lifestyle feature - *physical activity or the lack thereof*. I often wonder about the prevalence of chronic prostatitis globally 80 - 100 years ago compared to the present day. Based on limited epidemiological studies, we estimate a range from 5% to 15% of all men possibly suffer from prostatitis symptoms at least once in their lifetime. How many men suffered from prostatitis 100 years ago? We do not know. In the early half of the 20th century, prostatitis was attributed to buggy and horseback riding activities and also infections, especially connected to sexually transmitted infections such as gonorrhea.

In the modern era, gonorrhea is not as prevalent as it was 100 years ago, and we do not travel by buggy or horseback on a daily basis. Our technological advances have significantly impacted our lifestyle, especially our workplace lifestyle. I can tell you with certainty that in many years of dealing with chronic prostatitis patients, the overwhelming majority have had one common feature: sitting for work.

Here are the most common professions I encountered among our patients: computer related (IT, analysts, programmers, etc.), financial (bankers, accountants, etc.), lawyers, office clerks, drivers (trucks, taxis), and heavy machinery operators.

As you can see from the list above, there is one common denominator: they all have to sit long hours while working.

I assume there are more men, particularly in developed countries, who have to sit for long hours while working when compared to years ago. We need to clarify one thing here. Sitting is not responsible for causing an infection in the prostate. Men from all walks of life acquire infectious prostatitis regardless of what they do for a living.

Nevertheless, if we put infection aside, sitting definitely makes the symptoms of prostatitis worse.

Most men with CP report worsening of their symptoms closer to the end of the working day. If you spend a long time sitting, you will experience more symptoms. We do not exactly understand the mechanism of the action here. The assumption is that sitting will directly create more mechanical pressure on a prostate, which will make the gland more inflamed. Also, sitting will cause more pressure on the pelvic floor muscles and nerves. In time, the pelvic floor muscles will become stiffer, more inflamed and, therefore, cause more symptoms.

The most common symptom induced by sitting is pain. It is usually described as a dull, throbbing pain in the perineal (saddle) area ("golf ball" pressure), scrotum, upper thighs and lower back. In most of these cases we observe a mixed cause of this pain: prostate inflammation as well as stiff, inflamed perineal floor muscles. It is not uncommon to observe that men with CP who have had their prostate infection treated effectively still complain about sitting inducing symptoms. There is nothing unusual about this phenomenon.

I often use the following analogy: imagine an open wound somewhere on your skin which is in its healing phase. Instead of protecting it and allowing it to heal faster, you constantly chafe it or brush clothes against it. Obviously, it will take much longer to heal. The same principle applies to healing an inflamed prostate. Even if infection is no longer a factor, the prostate still remains inflamed for a while. In this case, prolonged sitting is like chafing a prostate along with surrounding tissues and muscles.

Prolonged sitting coupled with a stressful job usually complicates things even more.

I have heard it so many times. Men, under stress, with CP who do a lot of desk work feel pain on a higher level than their counterparts.

DEMYSTIFYING PROSTATITIS

Stress definitely triggers more pelvic floor muscles spasms, promotes more prostate inflammation and therefore increases pain.

It is almost universal that when I see my patients after at least a week-long vacation, they feel great. Once they start working their pain symptoms return.

What can we do about all this sitting? Unfortunately, there is no easy answer to this question. The good news is that men with infectious (i.e. bacteria, fungal) prostatitis feel better after appropriate treatment regardless of whether they sit for long periods or not. Nevertheless, there are men who will continue to feel symptoms related to sitting even after infection is no longer present.

Unfortunately, we cannot tell them to quit their desk jobs and go on a life-long vacation. I am sure it is a dream for most men with CP as it remains a dream for those without CP. We all have to work. So, we need to try to modify our sitting habits. My primary recommendation is to get up from your chair at least every 20-30 minutes and go for a fast walk somewhere. This walk might take just 1-2 minutes but does the job at achieving better blood flow to the pelvic floor area, creates a muscular workout, and takes the pressure off the prostate. Many of my patients argue that they go to the gym to exercise a few times per week. That is not enough. You need to keep moving throughout your working hours to minimize the negative impact of sitting.

You also need to pay attention to how you sit at work. If you lean forward while sitting, you apply more pressure on the affected area and are more likely to provoke inflammation and pain. In this case, I encourage men to lean back while sitting at their desks, be aware of pressure from your chair position, and try to modify it. Also recall my discussion in Chapter 4 about the importance of avoiding sitting on cold surfaces, how to amend that problem, and importance of wearing a long winter coat and warm boots during chilly winter months.

DEMYSTIFYING PROSTATITIS

By the way, I often wonder when watching western movies and see men sitting in recline position with their feet on a table: Does it have anything to do with their sore prostates from long horseback riding? After all, it comes down to the same thing, pressure on the perineal area.

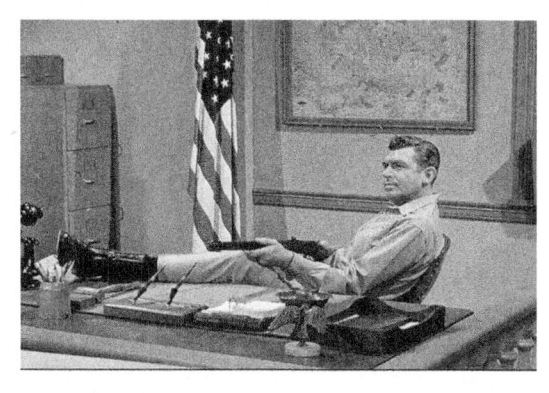

Unfortunately, it is much tougher when we advise men who are long haul truck drivers, or heavy machinery operators. They do not have the luxury of getting up every few minutes to go for a walk. You need to try to be creative here. Look at different seat cushions which will minimize the pressure and vibration emanating from your seats. Also, please remember, if you have a chance to get up and go for a quick walk, do it every time.

Lately, stand up desks have become popular in the workplace. Many companies these days even pay for them. Stand up desks allow the elimination of direct pressure on the perineal region. On the other hand, I still recommend that men who use stand up desks try to avoid standing still while working. Standing still can also promote stiffness in perineal muscles, along with venous blood stagnation in the region. No matter what, movement is a must. Even if you just wiggle your feet while standing, it's better than doing nothing.

What about exercise? As a rule, any type of exercise is good for you with, of course, some exceptions. Any type of exercise which requires sitting on a hard surface with the pressure on the perineal area, should be avoided. If you go to the gym, avoid upright stationary bicycles. Alternatively, you can use recumbent bikes, elliptical machines, or treadmills.

DEMYSTIFYING PROSTATITIS

If you like to lift weights, try to avoid using machines where you have to sit down. Otherwise, anything else is acceptable, especially free weights. Overall, when dealing with chronic prostatitis, we believe a cardio type of workout is better than weights. Also, any type of stretching is always encouraged. We definitely encourage you to do pelvic floor muscle stretching, yoga, tai chi, swimming or any other type of physical activity which boosts better blood flow to the perineal area along with muscular work out in this region.

But what if there's no way you're giving up cycling? There is nothing wrong with cycling as long as you modify your seat. If you feel a strong pressure in the perineal area while cycling, seat modification is a must. Often just adding extra padding to your seat does not solve the problem. Many men convert to specially designed seats where pressure on the perineum is totally eliminated. If you have a seat like that, and you feel no pain, there is no problem with cycling, and you can do it for as long as you want.

What about professional cyclists, the ones who do races? Their seats are typically narrow and hard. I am often compelled, when I drive along such a group of cyclists, to stretch my hand out and give them my business card. It is problematic. I honestly do not know if they are allowed to modify their seats. The least they can do is to push down the front part of the seat. This way the pressure may be redirected toward the bones of the pelvis on which you sit, not the perineal area. Moreover, it has been researched and published in medical peer reviewed journals that professional cyclists are more likely to suffer from erectile dysfunction due to the damage inflicted on the arteries supplying blood to the penile tissues. This damage emanates from the hard bicycle seat as well.

If you are the men who suffer from CP and are required to sit down for long hours, please try to follow the above recommendations. Regardless of what type of chronic prostatitis from which you suffer, regular physical activity and mobility will benefit not only your prostate, but your overall health.

DEMYSTIFYING PROSTATITIS

And so, we have reached the final part of this chapter:

Sexual behaviour

You can rightfully ask, "How does sexual behaviour have anything to do with lifestyle?"

I would argue that the way you conduct your sexual behaviour is a lifestyle choice. There is absolutely no doubt that sexual behaviour can have a direct impact on whether one person develops prostatitis and, also, whether it contributes to an inability to cure someone with prostatitis.

Let's be clear here. I am not going to discuss who you have sex with or how often. My main concern here is whether men subject themselves to a high risk of acquiring an infection through sexual contact. The infection, which can lodge itself in the prostate and lead to a typical chronic prostatitis condition, may take months and sometimes years to get rid of.

As you can see, sexual behaviour is a very relevant type of lifestyle which has direct implications in prostatitis development. It is an issue with young and sexually active single men. When men are in a long-term exclusive relationship, their risk of acquiring a bad infection through sex is less, compared to single men. Please be aware that having a steady partner does not necessarily prevent you from contracting infections. Women in general carry benign bacteria in their genital tract. Nonetheless, sometimes women develop a urinary tract infection, yeast infection, or present with nonspecific irritation, burning and occasional discharge, which may present as a case of bacterial vaginosis. If men have unprotected sex with their female partner during or around the time of such an occurrence, they subject themselves to a very high risk of acquiring the corresponding infection from their partner.

This infection can gradually find its way into the prostate and trigger prostatitis. It does not necessarily mean that men develop prostatitis shortly after exposure. The infection in the prostate may

DEMYSTIFYING PROSTATITIS

stay dormant (silent) for weeks, months and sometimes years. It often becomes "active" during a "perfect storm" when men's immune defences become weaker due to severe stress, sleep deprivation, bad dietary behaviour and/or a bad cold or flu.

The advice for men in steady relationships is to be aware of your partner's condition. If she claims to experience one of the above-mentioned problems, either abstain from sex all together until everything is completely clear or use condoms during sex.

If your partner is prone to UTI's or yeast infections and reports them quite often (i.e., more than 1-2 per year), condoms would be highly recommended.

We advise men who are sexually active with multiple partners that the use of condoms becomes vitally important. Firstly, your risk of acquiring a sexually transmitted infection (STI) becomes so much higher if you don't. What many men do not realize is that if they acquire some form of STI (e.g., gonorrhea, chlamydia), many other bacteria often enter the urethra along with the STI. You can eradicate an STI quite easily with prompt and appropriate antibiotics, but the other infection may remain intact. Again, gradually, it will find its way into the prostate and the risk of developing prostatitis becomes very high. Condoms are the only safety tool you have at your disposal.

Moreover, you should also be aware that receiving fellatio from a person who you barely know also puts you at high risk of acquiring some type of obscure infection via the introduction of various bacteria. It will not necessarily be a classic STI, but it can also cause urethritis and prostatitis. In this case, it is very difficult to recommend condoms, however, they may be used. You just have to weigh all the pros and cons of your behaviour and act accordingly.

There is another group of men who deserve special attention. Homosexual men, overall, suffer from prostatitis as often as heterosexual men. Some homosexual men may engage in higher risk sexual activities which puts them at a higher risk of acquiring different kinds of infections. In this case, only men who penetrate another person are at risk of developing prostatitis. If a man is on the receiving end and is in an exclusive relationship, there is minimal risk here. Please remember, infection has to enter the urethra in order to find its way into a person. The most common way this can occur is via anal penetration.

When men perform anal penetration without a condom, whether it be with a male or female partner, they are often exposed to all kinds of non-benign organisms. Therefore, the risk of bacterial prostatitis becomes very high. If you want to avoid such an ordeal, only condoms can save you.

On another note, regardless of sexual orientation, men who engage in penetrative sex, be it anally or orally, with multiple partners are at an extremely high risk of acquiring serious infections leading to prostatitis.

With the many men attending our clinic, I have seen all these scenarios. Everything I have described above is based on real cases.

It is up to you to decide who you want to have sex with and how, but please be aware of the potential risks out there and act sensibly.

I hope this chapter has not exhausted you too much. Please take a break, drink some water, go for a walk and move on to the next one.

CHAPTER 11

How expensive can pee really get?

This chapter is one of the most difficult and controversial chapters to discuss. The subject here are supplements (i.e., vitamins and herbal remedies). I remember about 25 years ago when vitamins and supplements were on the fringe of health care and health related topics in North America. Historically, herbal remedies have been used to treat different diseases for centuries. During the mid-19th century, treatment of many diseases was completely revolutionized due to significant advances in pharmacology.

In 1928, Dr. Alexander Fleming discovered penicillin, which changed our ability to fight bacterial infections and saved many lives. In 1921, a group of Canadian researchers invented insulin, which revolutionized the treatment of diabetes. In the 1940s, the first chemotherapy drugs were researched and developed. A new era of cancer treatment had begun, and thousands of people received a chance at beating an otherwise deadly disease.

These are a few examples of how research and development in pharmacology have changed the face of modern medicine. It is important to note that many of the drugs developed have an origin that stems from natural sources, such as plants. Examples of such drugs are aspirin (from willow bark), morphine (from opium poppy), scopolamine and atropine (from belladonna or deadly nightshade).

Many people believe that consumption of herbal remedies is completely harmless and that they can therefore consume countless

DEMYSTIFYING PROSTATITIS

amounts of herbal remedies in an attempt to receive some health benefit. In truth, this misguided practice can be as dangerous as the uncontrolled consumption of prescription drugs. Though many drugs originate from plants, most people don't realize that herbal remedies carry similar risks of overdose as do regular pharmaceutical drugs. They can be equally as toxic when consumed in excess, and in some cases even lethal. However, in the last few years, the popularity of herbal supplementation has grown substantially.

Traditional Chinese medicine is built on herbs. The Chinese have practiced herbal medicine for centuries and they have successfully treated many diseases by using herbs. Herbal medicine is embedded in their culture and built on knowledge and experience accumulated over centuries.

I, myself, grew up and practiced medicine in the former Soviet Union. I well remember that we also extensively used various herbal remedies in combination with traditional medicine for the treatment of colds, upper respiratory tract infections, arthritis and skin wound care. Russian folk medicine cannot be compared to Chinese medicine. It is not as advanced and does not have centuries of accumulated knowledge and experience. I personally had the impression that we used herbal remedies in practicing medicine due to a lack of access to drugs and medication. We simply had no drugs to recommend to our patients.

Now, the logical question arises; why have herbal remedies and supplements become so popular in North America?

For the last 20 years, I have treated men with prostatitis in Toronto. I have definitely noticed a significant increase in the use of herbal remedies over the last ten years. Certainly, there is no drug shortage and we cannot claim that the quality of drugs has declined either. So, what has made people turn to herbal supplements in western developed countries?

DEMYSTIFYING PROSTATITIS

It seems to me that it is due to a general trend toward a healthier lifestyle. There are more and more people who are more conscientious about eating healthier, being more physically active, and, overall, more health-oriented than ever before. Moreover, with climate change issues and environmental pollution affecting us globally, there are many more people who are turning towards herbal remedies as a healthy choice versus drugs, which many people see as chemicals poisoning our bodies.

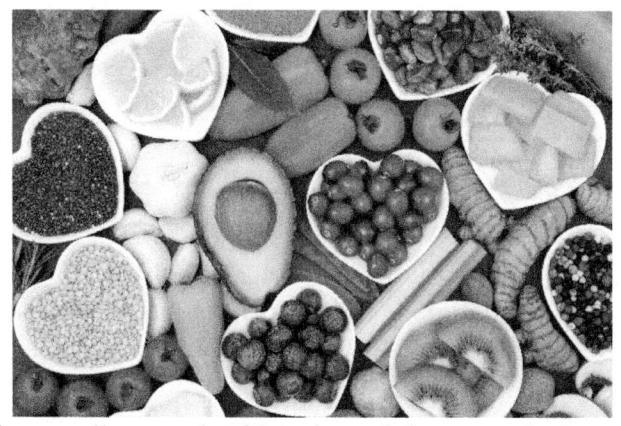

I have observed that many people these days are trying to establish a balance between taking medications and supplements to address their health needs. I do not have any problem with this approach. Even more so, I often utilize herbal supplements in management of chronic prostatitis. I believe that many herbal supplements have their role to play in helping men with CP.

Most of the patients I see for prostatitis are young men, aged 18-45. Though they are overall healthy individuals, many men disclose that they take either multivitamins, fish oil, omega-3 and more on a daily basis. When I ask them why they take these supplements, the standard reply is that they are supposed to be "good for you" because they possess antioxidant properties, and/or useful vitamins, minerals, etc. Some men appear to go to further extremes and take a very large number of different vitamins and supplements to support their various organs, glands and tissues specifically. Many of them take numerous supplements without having any relevant health issues. They take them just to potentially be healthier.

DEMYSTIFYING PROSTATITIS

Ironically, some of these men do not necessarily live a healthy lifestyle. They often consume processed foods, excess carbs and sugary products, and lack any amount of exercise. When I ask them how they feel, a typical response is "not so good". They usually complain about many health issues that they are still trying to control. I remember seeing one man in his forties who came to the office with a drug dispensing box filled with at least eight different supplements which were supposed to help him with his prostate, memory, adrenal glands, bones, stomach and God knows what else. He had many complaints to share about his health and he was not in high spirits. He was obviously not in a good state of health despite taking numerous supplements.

I would argue that taking too many supplements can be harmful for your health. It has been proven scientifically that you can practically poison yourself with overdosing on certain vitamins and minerals. Also, when various supplements are taken simultaneously, we do not know how they interact with each other. At the least, the effect of each supplement may diminish in effect. At the worst, the mixing of supplements can lead to the formation of toxic substances which can harm your health.

This approach to taking supplements is a completely wrong approach to healthy living.

We have already discussed healthy eating in the previous chapter. I am not going to repeat myself on this matter. The problem with supplements, especially vitamins, is that they are artificially produced. If you are a healthy person and you are not deficient in anything due to healthy eating habits, there is absolutely no reason for you to take multivitamins. Your body will simply not utilize them, will eliminate them and as a result you will certainly have the most expensive pee known to man.

I need to emphasize here that this notion applies to healthy individuals who live a healthy lifestyle. If you are a person with health problems and your doctor advises you to take certain supplements, it is a different ball game all together. You should definitely follow his/her advice.

Overall, we acquire essential microelements, minerals and vitamins from food products. They are much better absorbed and processed by our bodies when they are bonded with certain enzymes such as amino acids or fatty acids. On the contrary, in synthetic form, they are not processed unless we are deficient in some of these elements. That is why healthy eating is so much more valuable for your health than supplements.

So, the take home message is to please be thoughtful about taking supplements, especially when you are taking them because they are "good for your health." Do your homework, do your research, and see if healthy eating habits might be a much better alternative.

Further, I want to focus on supplements. I am not going to discuss them alone in detail because after all, this book is about prostatitis. So, I would like to discuss herbal remedies specifically designated for management of CP/CPPS.

It is not unusual for many men who suffer from CP/CPPS to search for herbal remedies in a quest to relieve their symptoms, especially when they go to specialty health food stores and face a dozen different supplements, all claiming to be good for the prostate. As a result, they face a dilemma in choosing which to use. They often rely on either the store clerk's recommendation or do an internet search to aid them in their decision making.

The truth is, if you carefully read the ingredients on the labels, there is at least a 60% overlap in each of their constituent ingredients. They actually only differ from each other in the brand and/or the actual company that makes them. I would like to remind you that herbal supplements are not drugs, and, therefore, they are not subjected to governmental oversight and control. As a result, the consumer simply relies on whether these manufactures really adhere

DEMYSTIFYING PROSTATITIS

to so-called GMP (Good Manufacturing Practices) and use high quality, raw materials obtained from, hopefully, reliable suppliers.

As you can see, we have a lot of "ifs" here before someone can be certain that they buy a good quality supplement. Unfortunately, we as consumers can only rely on brand names, claims, and possibly reviews in our purchasing decision making.

Another question arises: "Why do men with prostatitis need to use herbal supplements?"

Let me remind you that men who suffer from prostatitis suffer from chronic inflammation in the prostate. The actual word "prostatitis" means "inflamed prostate". The majority of herbal remedies recommended for "prostate" problems possess anti-inflammatory properties. That is the very essence of the herbal remedies' application in the case of chronic prostatitis. They are supposed to help minimize inflammation in the prostate gland. Whether they really work or not depends on many variables.

For example, if someone has a significant infection in the prostate, the supplements are highly unlikely to help. If someone has a significant neuromuscular problem within the pelvic floor around the prostate, supplements for the prostate will not help. Also, I have personally noticed a significant variation in men's response to different supplements. Some men claim a significant improvement with their symptoms while taking certain supplements, while on the contrary, other men have zero positive response to pretty much any supplement they have ever tried.

We should also be aware that supplements often carry a significant placebo effect (sugar pill effect). By the way, recent research on the placebo effect of drugs shows that it is beneficial for someone's health to experience a placebo effect. As far as I am concerned, if a certain supplement you take makes you feel better, go for it. Just make sure that you do not consume anything potentially harmful along the way.

DEMYSTIFYING PROSTATITIS

I often recommend certain supplements to my patients. Usually, I make these recommendations when my patients experience mild symptoms caused by low levels of inflammation. In some instances, I recommend supplements when my patients feel well but have some objective signs of inflammation within their prostate that remains present. I always measure my recommendations against individuals' perception and attitude towards supplements and their overall lifestyle. A healthy lifestyle always trumps supplements. If someone is a poor eater (consumes lots of junk food, sugary drinks, beer, etc.) taking a shelf full of supplements will do nothing for him. Please remember, a healthy lifestyle is your priority. Everything else is secondary.

I am assuming some of you would like to know which herbal supplements I would recommend for chronic prostatitis.

First of all, I am not going to mention any particular brands. It may be perceived that I promote them through my book. I am simply going to list a few herbal remedies that I know can potentially have an anti-inflammatory effect on the prostate. It is fair to mention that there are only a limited number of herbal supplements which have been researched to a certain degree and proven scientifically to have some anti-inflammatory effect on the prostate specifically.

They are:
- Saw Palmetto (Serenoa Repens)
- Cernilton (Flower Pollen Extract)
- Quercetin
- Pygeum Africanum (raw material is no longer available in true form).

These are the only herbal remedies that have some limited scientific data to support their anti-inflammatory effect on the prostate. The following long list of other herbal remedies possess systemic anti-inflammatory and antioxidant properties and therefore,

DEMYSTIFYING PROSTATITIS

often become part of a multi-ingredient composition of many supplements currently sold on the market.

The main ingredients are:
- Garlic
- Turmeric
- Zinc
- Beta Sitosterol
- Ginger
- Ginseng
- Cranberry extract
- Pumpkin seeds
- Stinging Nettle
- Green tea leaf.

This list is by no means exhaustive. There are many natural products such as herbs, fruits and vegetables that claim to possess antioxidant properties, which means they also have an anti-inflammatory effect. That is why it is essential to have them incorporated in your regular dietary habits. Whether they are as effective when you take them in supplemental form still remains the subject of debate. I think a lot depends on the quality of the supplement manufacturing and the individuals' response.

Not every person responds well to supplements. There are men who experience side effects from taking certain supplements, such as stomach upsets and allergic reactions. You also have to be cautious about taking supplements along with other medications, both over the counter and prescription. It is always advisable to inform your doctor and your pharmacist about any supplements you are taking when you intend to take a drug.

Here, we have reached the end of this chapter. What I was trying to say here is, if you really need to take certain vitamins or herbal remedies due to specific health problems, you should try them for some time. After taking them for a period of about 2-3 months, you should assess whether you indeed feel better specifically because you have taken these specific vitamins or supplements. If there is no change in the way you feel, most likely these certain vitamins/supplements have done nothing for you and, therefore, there is no reason to take them further.

It is always advisable to consult with your health provider and/or naturopathic specialist if you experience difficulty deciding whether you should take any supplement or which one you should take. You should also be very careful when taking too many supplements at the same time. If you end up taking more than two or three supplements, you should seriously examine the necessity of taking at least some of them. Even more so, if you also take prescription medications simultaneously, you should definitely consult your health care provider and/or pharmacist.

If you take certain vitamins/supplements just because they are supposed to be "good for you", it is time to ditch them into a trash collector.

Please remember, a healthy lifestyle such as healthy eating, healthy liquid consumption, staying physically active daily and getting a good night's sleep are your main vitamins and supplements. Everything else should be considered only if you really need them and a healthy lifestyle is not enough to maintain your good health.

That is all, my dear readers. We have reached the end of this chapter, but also the end of this story.

There is only the Conclusion left to go through. I really hope that it is going to be shorter than any chapter. Please be a good sport and read it.

But, if you feel quite tired right now, put this book aside and have something nice to eat and drink, or go for a pleasant walk. Hopefully, I will meet you again soon at the finish line...

DEMYSTIFYING PROSTATITIS

IN CONCLUSION

Do I get used to it or Do something about it?

Finally, we have reached the end of the prostate story. When I look back at the chapters I've written, it seems the book is not that big. There are much bigger books out there written on different subjects: fiction, non-fiction, mysteries, murders, health, romance and life. My book cannot, of course, compete with "War and Peace" by Leo Tolstoy. Honestly, when I was writing this book, it was never my intention to overwhelm you with too much information. I believe that most men, including myself, have a short attention span, especially in our modern era of busy lives, already overloaded with too much information coming from TV, computers and social media. I wanted my book to present the information which would be the most relevant to men who either suffer from Chronic Prostatitis or are yet to develop this condition.

The reality of mankind is that every boy has a prostate. As we males mature, and especially when we enter the post-puberty stage, our prostate becomes a target for infection and inflammation. I hope I've reflected these risk factors in my chapter on foreskin and circumcision.

When men become sexually active, the risk factors for developing an infection in the prostate double and even triple. Young, single men who are involved in unprotected sexual behaviour with random partners are risking their prostate health every time they're out there.

What I am saying is that this book is intended for all men, regardless of whether you have prostatitis or not. I think that this book MUST be read by all men of all ages.

If you are a young man with a completely healthy prostate, you should read this book. It will provide you with knowledge about how

DEMYSTIFYING PROSTATITIS

to live your life, so you minimize the risks of developing chronic prostatitis. If you are a man who suffers from chronic prostatitis, hopefully this book will help you learn how to alleviate at least some of the symptoms of prostatitis and make your life more manageable.

If you are a much older man who suffers from symptoms of prostate enlargement (BPH), this book may help you as well. It has been scientifically proven that a worsening of BPH related symptoms are often caused by prostate inflammation or infection (i.e. chronic prostatitis).

There is only one category of men for whom this book will be least helpful, and they are men who have had their prostate removed for prostate cancer. Unfortunately, in this case, it is already too late to help. But if you are a man with very localized prostate cancer and not being treated for it, this book is worth reading. There are a lot of men who have very localized prostate cancer and prostatitis at the same time. I hope this book will help you too.

The whole focus of my book was on educating men about prostatitis. I want you to know what prostatitis and Chronic Pelvic Pain Syndrome is about. I want you to understand why men develop prostatitis and what factors can make it worse.

I have, in this book, done a considerable amount of writing regarding lifestyle. I believe that lifestyle is one of the cornerstones of developing, or not developing, prostatitis in the first place. But also, lifestyle often has a significant impact on how men with prostatitis feel symptomatically. In many men, just some simple lifestyle modifications have led to complete resolution of prostatitis symptoms and eventual cure.

The purpose of this book has been to educate men about the prostate and prostatitis as being one of the most common diseases of the prostate. I want men to be empowered with this knowledge. Everything that I have written in this book can be controlled by men themselves.

DEMYSTIFYING PROSTATITIS

You are in control of your lifestyle, sexual behaviour, dietary habits and herbal supplementation if you deem it necessary.

What you cannot control is how you are being treated. If you are a man with all the signs and symptoms of chronic prostatitis, there is a good chance that you are going to see your General Practitioner and possibly a Urologist. Many of you might have seen your doctor more than once. You have no control over what your doctor prescribes, if anything. Obviously, it is up to a physician to decide what medication he or she would recommend you use at that particular moment. That is why I have avoided any medical recommendations.

Chronic Prostatitis/Chronic Pelvic Pain Syndrome is a very complex condition. It entails different kinds of infection, which are often very challenging to diagnose. It comprises inflammation, muscular and possibly neurogenic problems in a pelvic area.

Every man who suffers from this condition is unique. He is unique in the underlying cause of his condition. He is unique in terms of the other factors which can influence how his case of prostatitis responds to one or another treatment. He is also unique in terms of lifestyle, which, as we know, can also have an impact on this condition.

As you can see, every man is a brand-new case which requires a very personalized assessment and treatment. There is no structured protocol for assessment and treatment. There are guidelines, but they are generic and might be helpful only for urologists, who have a stronger interest in managing prostatitis patients. As a matter of fact, most men who suffer from CP/CPPS are managed by their General Practitioners whom you can not expect to be specialists on prostatitis.

These are the reasons why I tried to write on how to diagnose and treat prostatitis. Every doctor out there is on their own. Unfortunately, there are only a handful of clinics which specialize in this field. I can not simply write in this book what I would do as a practitioner and expect you to get the same approach from any physician. Let me remind you again: every man who suffers from CP/CPPS is unique

DEMYSTIFYING PROSTATITIS

and therefore each man's treatment should be unique and specific to him. General advice may not be as effective as treatment tailored to each individual case.

If you are in need of medical attention, I really hope that you are in luck and the doctor you see understands you and understands your problem.

I wish you all the best in your lives. I wish you a normal-size, healthy and happy prostate.

I hope that you enjoyed reading this book. It's not a big one but contains everything you need to know. You can put it in your backpack, you can put it under your pillow or keep it in your glove compartment. I hope that you utilize this book as a resource to which you can refer whenever you need it.

So long my dear readers!

Now it is time to do a few sit ups and go for a long healthy walk.

Cheers!

ACKNOWLEDGEMENTS

Harvey Brownstone, more than a friend. You are certainly a part of our family. The very idea of writing this book was conceived in the basement of your house. You managed to secure it in my mind despite my unrelenting scepticism and whining. You inspired me to work on this project and proved to me that I can do it. Your passion and trust in what I do were at the roots of this work. I am also incredibly grateful for all the editing and ideas you put forward. Your help with work on this book was indispensable to me.

Steve Silver, friend, and advisor to my book project. Your help with book editing, formatting, and image design, was amazing. I cannot imagine how I could have finished this project without your help.

Hanna Kaploun, my daughter. You were among the first to cheer me into writing this book. You have suffered through first line editing. I am sorry that you had to put up with my command of the written English language and my annoyance with at times being misunderstood. But you were patient and kind with me. I am eternally grateful for all you hard work.

Kristen Kaploun, my daughter-in-law, Doctor of Clinical Psychology. Despite your remarkably busy professional life and being a mom of two beautiful girls, our grand daughters, you have found time to proofread my book and polish it to perfection. I am so grateful for your support and time spent working on my book. If I ever write another book, consider yourself hired.

Maxim Kaploun, my son, and hard-working attorney. I am grateful for your encouragement, for you believing in me. Also, I am grateful for the legal counsel your provided to help with launching my book. Your legal expertise is very much appreciated.

DEMYSTIFYING PROSTATITIS

Joe and Lauren, friends, and family to us. We have been close friends for many years. Throughout years of hardship as new immigrants to Canada, your friendship was invaluable to me. You were one of the few people at the onset of my medical career in Canada who supported me and my family every step of the way. Our numerous conversations about prostate health have helped me to shape many chapters in this book. Your enthusiasm and encouragement helped me to keep writing this book to the end regardless how busy or tired I was.

Finally, last but not at all least, is my wife Luba. I do not even know where to begin. We have been together for almost 40 years now. We have lived through dark times and happy times. You have always looked at me as one who knows it all when it comes to medicine. Even in our darkest times you always believed that I would rise again and continue my professional journey in helping others. You are the love of my life. Without your inspiration, without your unconditional love and support, this book would never have been written. You are my staunchest critic and greatest admirer. Thank you for standing by me through all these years. I am humbled and honoured to have you by my side.

REFERENCES

1. John N. Krieger, Shaun Wen Huey Lee, Jeonseong Jeon, Phaik Yeong Cheah, Men Long Liong, and Donald E. Riley. Epidemiology of prostatitis. Int J Antimicrob Agents. 2008 Feb; 31(Suppl 1): S85–S90.

2. Paul J Turek, MD; Chief Editor: Jeter (Jay) Pritchard Taylor III, MD. Prostatitis (Epidemiology). Medscape Updated: Nov 01, 2019

3. Tripp DA1, Nickel JC, Ross S, Mullins C, Stechyson N. Prevalence, symptom impact and predictors of chronic prostatitis-like symptoms in Canadian males aged 16-19 years. BJU Int. 2009 Apr;103(8):1080-4.

4. Fusco F, Arcaniolo D, Restaino A, Lauri I, Franzese C. Prevalence of chronic prostatic inflammation based on clinical diagnostic criteria in a real practice setting: a nation-wide observational study. SIUT Prostatic Inflammation Study Group. Minerva Urol Nefrol. 2017 Oct;69(5):509-518.

5. Collins MM, Stafford RS, O'Leary MP, Barry MJ. How common is prostatitis? A national survey of physician visits. J Urol. 1998; 159:1224–8.

6. SM Orland, PM Hanno, AJ Wein. Prostatitis, prostatosis, and prostatodia. Urology, 1985 – Elsevier.

7. JJ Stevermer, SK Easley. Treatment of prostatitis. American family physician, 2000.

8. JN Krieger, L Nyberg Jr, JC Nickel. NIH consensus definition and classification of prostatitis Jama, 1999, 282(3):236-237.

9. AJ Schaeffer. Classification (traditional and National Institutes of Health) and demographics of prostatitis. Urology, Volume 60, Issue 6, Supplement, December 2002, Pages 5-6.

10. Jon Rees, Mark Abrahams, Andrew Doble, Alison Cooper, and the Prostatitis Expert Reference Group (PERG). Diagnosis and treatment of chronic bacterial prostatitis and chronic prostatitis/chronic pelvic pain syndrome: a consensus guideline. BJU Int. 2015 Oct; 116(4): 509–525.

11. Zegarra Montes LZ, Sanchez Mejia AA, Loza Munarriz CA, Gutierrez EC. Semen and urine culture in the diagnosis of chronic bacterial prostatitis. Int Braz J Urol. 2008 Jan-Feb;34(1):30-7, discussion 38-40.

12. Krieger JN, Riley DE. Prostatitis: what is the role of infection. Int J Antimicrob Agents 2002, Jun;19(6):475-9.

13. DA Shoskes, J Altemus, AS Polackwich, B Tucky et al. Analysis of Gut Microbiome Reveals Significant Differences between Men with Chronic Prostatitis/Chronic Pelvic Pain Syndrome and Controls. Urology, Volume 92, June 2016, Pages 26-32.

14. Aragón IM, Herrera-Imbroda B et al. The Urinary Tract Microbiome in Health and Disease. Eur Urol Focus. 2018 Jan;4(1):128-138.

15. Alwithanani et al., Periodontal Treatment Improves Prostate Symptoms and Lowers Serum PSA in Men with High PSA and Chronic Periodontitis. Dentistry 2015, 5:3.

16. Andre Paes B da Silva, Leela Subhashini C Alluri et al. Association between oral pathogens and prostate cancer: building the relationship. Am J Clin Exp Urol. 2019; 7(1): 1–10.

17. Mary McNaughton Collins, MD, MPH, Michel A Pontari, MD, Michael P O'Leary, MD et al, and The Chronic Prostatitis Collaborative Research Network. Quality of Life Is Impaired in Men with Chronic Prostatitis. J Gen Intern Med. 2001 Oct; 16(10): 656–662.

18. Tripp DA, Curtis Nickel J, Landis JR, Wang YL, Knauss JS; CPCRN Study Group. Predictors of quality of life and pain in chronic prostatitis/chronic pelvic pain syndrome: findings from the National Institutes of Health Chronic Prostatitis Cohort Study. BJU Int. 2004 Dec;94(9):1279-82.,

19. Wenninger K Heiman JR, Rothman I, Berghuis JP, Berger RE. Sickness impact of chronic nonbacterial prostatitis and its correlates. The Journal of Urology, 29 Feb 1996, 155(3):965-968.

20. KU JH, Kim ME, Lee NK, Park YH. Influence of environmental factors on chronic prostatitis-like symptoms in young men: results of a community-based survey. Urology, 30 Nov 2001, 58(6):853-858.

21. Anthony J. Schaeffer, J. Richard Landis, Jill S. Knauss, Kathleen J. Propert, Richard B. Alexander, Mark S. Litwin, J. Curtis Nickel, Michael P. O'Leary, Robert B. Nadler, Michel A. Pontari, Daniel A. Shoskes, Scott I. Zeitlin, Jackson E. Fowler, Carissa A. Mazurick, Lori Kishel, John W. Kusek. Demographic and Clinical Characteristics of Men with Chronic Prostatitis: The National Institutes of Health Chronic Prostatitis Cohort Study. The Journal of Urology, August 2002, Volume 168, Issue 2, Pages 593-598.

22. Oleg Banyra, Olha Ivanenko, Oleg Nikitin, and Alexander Shulyak. Mental status in patients with chronic bacterial prostatitis. Cent European J Urol. 2013; 66(1): 93–100.

23. Riegel B, Bruenahl CA, Ahyai S, Bingel U, Fisch M, Löwe B. Assessing psychological factors, social aspects and psychiatric co-morbidity associated with Chronic Prostatitis/Chronic Pelvic Pain Syndrome (CP/CPPS) in men -- a systematic review. J Psychosom Res. 2014 Nov;77(5):333-50.

24. Nickel JC, Tripp DA, Chuai S, et al. Psychosocial variables affect the quality of life of men diagnosed with chronic prostatitis/chronic pelvic pain syndrome. BJU Int. 2008;101(1):59-64.

25. Lim KB. Epidemiology of clinical benign prostatic hyperplasia. Asian J Urol. 2017 Jul;4(3):148-151.

26. Patel ND, Parsons JK. Epidemiology and etiology of benign prostatic hyperplasia and bladder outlet obstruction. Indian J Urol. 2014 Apr;30(2):170-6.

27. Nickel JC. Inflammation and benign prostatic hyperplasia. Urol Clin North Am. 2008;35(1):109.

28. Brenner DR, Weir HK, Demers AA, Ellison LF, Louzado C, Shaw A, Turner D, Woods RR, Smith LM. Projected estimates of cancer in Canada in 2020, CMAJ. 2020;192: E199-205.

29. St Sauver JL, Jacobson DJ, McGree ME, Girman CJ, Lieber MM, Jacobsen SJ. Longitudinal association between prostatitis and development of benign prostatic hyperplasia. Urology. 2008;71(3):475-479.

30. Delongchamps NB, de la Roza G, Chandan V, et al. Evaluation of prostatitis in autopsied prostates--is chronic inflammation more associated with benign prostatic hyperplasia or cancer? J Urol. 2008;179(5):1736-1740.

31. Projected estimates of cancer in Canada in 2020. Darren R. Brenner, Hannah K. Weir, Alain A. Demers, Larry F at al. CMAJ Mar 2020, 192 (9) E199-E205.

Printed in Great Britain
by Amazon